Measuring
psychopathology

Measuring psychopathology

ANNE FARMER
PETER McGUFFIN
JULIE WILLIAMS

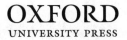

OXFORD
UNIVERSITY PRESS

OXFORD

UNIVERSITY PRESS

Great Clarendon Street, Oxford OX2 6DP

Oxford University Press is a department of the University of Oxford.
It furthers the University's objective of excellence in research, scholarship,
and education by publishing worldwide in

Oxford New York

Athens Auckland Bangkok Bogotá Bombay Buenos Aires Calcutta
Cape Town Dar es Salaam Delhi Florence Hong Kong Istanbul
Karachi Kuala Lumpur Madrid Melbourne Mexico City Mumbai
Nairobi Paris São Paulo Shanghai Singapore Taipei Tokyo Toronto Warsaw

and associated companies in Berlin Ibadan

Published in the United States
by Oxford University Press Inc., New York

First published 2002

British Library Cataloguing in Publication Data

Data available

Library of Congress Cataloging in Publication Data

ISBN 0 19 263080 6

10 9 8 7 6 5 4 3 2 1

Typeset by TechBooks, India
Printed on acid-free paper by Biddles Ltd, Guildford & King's Lynn

Contents

CHAPTER 1

....

What is
Psychopathology?

Introduction

Consider this question. Have you worried a lot over the past month? Answering 'yes' may indicate that you are just experiencing normal concern about the usual tribulations of life. Alternatively, your worrying may be an indicator that you have a mental disorder. Establishing whether worrying is a symptom of a psychiatric disorder, or merely a normal experience, requires answers to a number of supplementary questions such as 'What's it like when you worry?' 'Can you turn your attention to anything else?' and 'How much of the time over the past month have you worried?' When worrying becomes a recurrent and painful round of thoughts, so that it is difficult to turn your attention to anything else and takes up much of your time, then your worrying is more likely to be a symptom of a mental disorder (Wing *et al.* 1974).

Knowing what supplementary questions to ask and their significance allows the rater to determine whether worrying is pathological or not. The answers relating to worrying will also prompt questions about other symptoms which may be associated with worrying, such as nervous tension, low mood and anxiety. By careful cross-examination undertaken in a systematic way, the skilled rater can build up a picture of the mental experiences of the respondent (Wing *et al.* 1974). Such enquiry will include questions regarding experiences of anxiety, such as panic, phobias, and obsessions, mood-states such as depression or mania, sleep and appetite disturbances, bodily aches and pains, and abnormal experiences such as hearing voices and having false beliefs. These abnormal symptoms and signs are further discussed in chapter 2.

This process also incorporates an attempt to arrive at an objective judgement about the nature and severity of each symptom. For example, although, you could tick a box on a questionnaire to indicate that you had worried a lot, but this would only indicate your *subjective* view of your worrying. As we shall discuss later, (particularly in chapter 7 on rating scales, chapter 8 on psychopathology in specific subject groups, and chapter 9 on personality and personality disorders) questionnaires have an important role in assessing psychopathology. However, this is rather different from the role of face to face interviews that include the type of careful enquiry described above, whereby the degree and severity of individual symptoms is weighed up.

Mental disorders are defined according to the clustering together of various subjective complaints or symptoms and observable abnormalities in behaviour, cognition or speech (signs) which are considered to be pathological. Such clusters of signs and symptoms are termed syndromes, and to date there are no objective tests available which can confirm or refute their presence. Eliciting pathological symptoms is dependent on those with the symptoms being able to articulate and communicate their experiences and on the researcher or clinician being sufficiently empathic to understand and interpret their significance. This interaction between sufferer and observer also depends on what is considered pathological in the culture(s) to which they both belong, which, in turn, may be influenced by language, education, religious beliefs or politics. Assessing psychopathology, which can be defined as *the study of abnormal states of mind*, is the key to this process.

The system of clinical enquiry that we have outlined above is the main method clinicians use to elicit psychopathology. Having determined what pathological features are present, it is then possible to assign the individual to a diagnostic category. In the clinical setting, diagnosis is assigned by a clinician who attempts to match the symptom profile of the subject to a 'mental template' acquired through clinical experience. This mental template is derived from groups of individuals who share psychopathological features in common. For example, the clinician may decide that the person's psychopathology most resembles those who have schizophrenia rather than those who have bipolar disorder. Therefore the most likely diagnosis is schizophrenia.

As we will describe later (see chapters 3 and 4) this approach has led to much inconsistency and a lack of agreement between clinicians, so more structured and reliable methods have been devised to improve diagnostic accuracy, and these are particularly applicable for research. One such approach is to use computerized scoring programs to assign a diagnostic category or categories, free from any human error or prejudices on behalf of the clinician (Kramer 1961, Wing *et al.* 1974, McGuffin *et al.* 1991) (see also chapter 6). In addition, the clinical enquiry method has been systematized into structured and semi-structured interviews which has helped to improve the reliability of diagnosis (Robins *et al.* 1981, Wing *et al.* 1990). These are further described in chapter 5.

The approach we have outlined above, using 'worrying' as an example, is termed *phenomenological psychopathology*. The process we have detailed relates to objective descriptions of morbid mental experiences or *phenomena* and does not rely on any theories about what may have caused them. Phenomenological psychopathology is also concerned with the empathic understanding of conscious experiences and observable behaviour, described by Jaspers (1963) as *'representing, defining and classifying psychic phenomena as an independent activity'*.

There are two other principal approaches to the assessment of psychopathology. First, *psychodynamic* psychopathology was derived from psychoanalytic theory, where it is proposed that unconscious mental processes generate abnormal mental events. Unlike phenomenological psychopathology, which examines the abnormal phenomena in detail, psychodynamic psychopathology mainly concentrates on the unconscious mechanisms (e.g. repression, projection) that are assumed to have caused them. Second, *experimental* psychopathology concerns the testing of hypotheses regarding the relationships between normal experiences and abnormal mental events. It includes a broad range of research methods, including using animal models of human behaviour.

The main focus in this book is on descriptive and phenomenological psychopathology, together with the various methods that can be used to enhance the reliability and validity of measurement. In addition, some of the approaches that we will discuss also draw upon experimental psycho-pathological methods (see chapters 8 and 9). The researcher who is not a clinician may be baffled by all this concern with the importance of the mea-surement of psychopathology and not wish to get involved in this aspect of the research. Indeed, it may well seem preferable just to leave the 'diagnosis' entirely to clinical collaborators. In the following chapters, we will outline why this may lead to unsatisfactory research findings and will stress the im-portance of paying careful attention to the evaluation of psychopathology.

Attempts to categorize mental disorders have been made at least since the times of the ancient Greeks. To understand the current 'state of play', regarding the classification of mental disorders, it is important to briefly examine some historical developments.

The development of a scientific approach to the measurement of psychopathology

Modern scientific thinking about the measurement of psychopathology has developed via two main paradigms, described by Kendler (1990) as 'the great professor principle' and the 'consensus of experts'. Over the past three centuries, psychiatrists from different European countries developed their own classifications (or *nosologies*) of mental disorders. These were influenced by prevailing philosophies and beliefs relating to the insane, the doctors' own opinions as well as their examinations of the patients in their charge. Some of the eminent men who shaped ideas about psycho-pathology during the nineteenth and early twentieth centuries included Pinel, Esquirol, Falret, Magnan, Morel and Charcot in France, Bucknill, Tuke, Maudsley and Pritchard in the UK, and Reil, Heinroth, Griesinger, Kahlbaum, Hecker, Kraepelin and Schneider in Germany. Those they taught then promulgated their professor's diagnostic system throughout the local area, region or country. Clearly, some of these famous professors had more influence than others. However, there were many different competing nosologies, even within the same country, but very few of these enjoyed a more general acceptance.

One notable exception to this lack of general applicability of the 'grand professorial' classifications was that proposed by Emil Kraepelin, (1856–1926) a German psychiatrist who meticulously examined patients over many years. In the 1890s he devised a system of collecting, sorting and comparing information on groups of patients on cards. It is still a matter of debate as to whether he derived his nosological system from the results of his card sorting methods, or whether he simply used these data to support a classification scheme based on his clinical intuitions. Which ever is the case his approach to classification, published in the fifth edition of his textbook in 1896 had, and continues to have, considerable influence regarding the main divisions and categories of mental disorder. Kraepelin's approach was arguably more scientific than any of his contemporaries or predecessors. He carefully observed not just the pattern of his patients' symptoms and but also their course over time. He attempted to discover common features in the psychopathology that both distinguished between groups and would be of value in assessing *prognosis* (i.e. the outcome of the disorder over time). On the basis of his careful cross sectional, plus longitudinal observations, he was able to classify mental disorders into three main classes, the organic psychoses (where structural brain abnormalities could be shown), the endogenous psychoses (where structural pathology could not be demonstrated) and deviations of the personality and reactive states. The main Kraeplinian categories and the types of disorder that are contained in each (using modern terminology) are listed in table 1.1. Among the strengths and novelty of Kraepelin's approach was its potential, in his view, to help to discover the cause of mental disorders, and to classify these by their causation (*aetiology*). Subsequently prevention and treatment could be based on this *aetiological* knowledge.

In the second half of the twentieth century the 'consensus of experts' paradigm took over, and official nosologies for national and international use were developed (Kendler 1990) (see also chapter 3). In this approach, national and international bodies convened committees of expert in order to produce the classifications. Various criteria were employed to make decisions about the constituent elements of the diagnostic categories, such as current diagnostic practice, historical perspective, and personal clinical opinion, as well as what research evidence was available at the time. As the research base relating to mental disorders developed, there was an increasing amount of objective evidence on which to base the classification. Probably the largest shift in thinking and practice took place as a result of the *Diagnostic and Statistical Manual,* third edition (DSMIII), published by the American Psychiatric Association in 1980.

The DSMIII classification has been a watershed in the modern approach to the classification of mental disorders. Not only was the *scientific evidence* the main guiding principle for the expert panel, but also a new system of

Table 1.1 Kraepelin's main categories of mental disorder.

	Organic psychosis	Endogenous psychosis	Deviations of the personality and reactive states
Defining features	Loss of contact with reality, demonstrable brain pathology or metabolic disturbance	Loss of contact with reality, no demonstrable pathology or metabolic disturbance	Contact with reality preserved
Examples using modern nomenclature	Dementia, e.g. Alzheimer's Disease, multi-infarct dementia Confusional states, e.g. delerium tremens	Schizophrenia, Bipolar affective disorder Unipolar depressive disorder with psychotic features (delusions or hallucinations)	Unipolar depressive disorder Generalized anxiety disorder Obsessive compulsive disorder All personality disorders (axis II of DSM IV)

defining mental disorders was introduced for the first time to a national nosology. This new system was the use of explicit or *operational criteria* to define the categories of mental disorder. Although now universally accepted, when introduced initially for research purposes, defining mental disorders using this operationalized approach was a radical approach. The use of operational definitions for the first time in a national classification was even more so: thus, the publication of DSMIII represented a real paradigm shift in the definition of mental disorders. Although there have been subsequent classifications since DSMIII, these more recent publications employ the same general approach. We will further consider the role of operational criteria in defining mental disorders in chapters 3 and 4.

Alternative views: Freud and Meyer

We have already mentioned the psychodynamic (or psychoanalytic) approach to psychopathology, which examines the unconscious mechanisms believed to underlie abnormal mental experiences. Psychodynamic theory was largely the creation of Sigmund Freud (1856–1939), an almost exact contemporary of Kraepelin. The psychoanalytic theories of Freud have had, and continue to have, an enormous influence beyond psychiatry and psychology in offering explanations of both normal and pathological mental life. The beginning of Freudian theory derived from his original observations published in 1895 (just a year before Kraepelin published his landmark fifth edition of his textbook) and were based on the treatment of a hysterical patient by the use of hypnosis (Freud 1895). These early observations led to Freud's conception of the unconscious, as well as his notion of 'repression'. Freud's main tenet was that the emotion attached to repressed memories could affect the individual's response to events in the present. From these beginnings Freud and his followers constructed the great edifice of psychodynamic theory that exerted a looming influence over psychiatry in most of the United States and large tracts of Western Europe for much of the mid twentieth century. Freud, of course, remains the most prominent and famous of psychopathologists in the minds of educated lay persons, and his theories are still influential in art, literature and in certain strands of popular psychology. His notions about what takes place in the psychotherapeutic process continue to have wide currency among psychiatrists, clinical psychologists and other therapists. However, almost nowhere is Freudian theory seen as part of the main stream in the study of psychopathology.

A detailed consideration of why this is the case is beyond our scope. However we offer two possible and partly overlapping explanations. The first is that the psychodynamic approach to psychopathology does not easily open itself to scientific scrutiny, or generate hypotheses that are testable by empirical methods. Therefore psychoanalytic methods look increasingly unattractive in an era that demands objectivity, and where there is increasing support for evidence-based clinical practice. The second, perhaps more subtle reason for a decline in confidence in Freudian ideas has been the realization, first articulated by Jaspers (1963), that psychodynamic theory appears to offer *causal explanations* of thought and behaviour, but in actuality only provides *meaningful connections* concerning the ways in which mental states arise. For example, classical Freudian theory sees obsessional traits of orderliness, parsimony and obstinacy as arising out of a 'fixation' at the anal stage of development when the individual was being potty trained. While the concept of an 'anal retentive' trait provides a nice metaphor that might help somewhat in understanding the thought processes of the stubborn, obsessive-compulsive hand-washer, it strains credulity to suggest that some aspect of his toilet training was *a cause* of his illness.

A figure who enjoyed much less popular fame but who was also a highly influential teacher of psychiatry was Adolf Meyer (1866–1950). He founded a *psychobiological* school of thought regarding psychopathology (Meyer 1957). Meyer and his followers considered that the individual was unique, and that it was not desirable to break this unity into several aspects, or to classify it into a category of simple disease entities. He regarded mental disorder as a psychobiological reaction that involved both physical and mental aspects, immediate stress and/or past habits of adjustment. The main features of Meyer's philosophy were the unity of body and mind, the uniqueness of the individual, and the necessary combination of psychological and biological aspects in the causation of mental disorder. He taught that the concept of disease entities was at best misleading, and at worst illusory, and instead proposed that abnormal mental states be described as *reaction types*. That is, it is preferable not to subscribe to the existence of disorders such as schizophrenia or depression, but only to schizophrenic or depressive reaction types. Meyer also introduced the idea of a *'formulation'* for each case. He stated that it was

> Possible to formulate the main facts of most cases in terms of a natural chain of cause and effect, utilizing the psychobiological material at hand, better than a dogmatic assumption of a specific but hypothetically unitary toxic principle.

The idea that the salient clinical features of a case are better presented as a formulation or summary assessment rather that just a bald diagnosis is fairly widely accepted but, as with Freud, the influence of Meyer has faded considerably. However, it remains the case that we understand little about the causes of most psychopathology, despite the technological and pharmacological advances of the past two decades. Consequently, there are still those who question the need to classify mental disorders. Therefore, we will consider the arguments against and in favour of categorizing psychopathology.

Why classify? The case against

We have already said that at the present time most psychopathological signs and symptoms cannot be verified by any biological tests: therefore their presence can be considered merely a matter of opinion, which calls into question issues of reliability and validity. The case has been made (Szasz 1962) that the mental events which are defined as abnormal are produced by the mind. Since the mind is not an organ of the body, it cannot be diseased in the same way as it is possible for the body to be diseased. That is, the mind cannot show demonstrable pathology or *lesions*. The obvious answer to this criticism is that surely the mind must be 'located' in the brain. Although it remains true that few pathological abnormalities can be shown in those experiencing mental disorders, it is argued that this is because the brain abnormalities are subtle and the technologies which can identify them have not yet been developed. Clearly the argument can become a philosophical one. You either *believe* that mental disorders are produced by as yet unidentified alterations in brain structure and function, or you do not. Other critics of the medical model have gone further and have stated that mental disorders are hypothetical constructs, and that rather than talk about 'illness' or 'disease', it would be better to discuss maladaptive behaviour, communication difficulties, or problems with living (Scheff 1966, Erikson 1964).

However, although there have been vigorous proponents of a 'disease free' approach to psychopathology over several decades, this has inevitably led to chaos and confusion. There has not been one consistent and testable alternative hypothesis that has been proposed regarding the nature of mental disorders. It is as if de-medicalizing the measurement of psycho-pathology leads to a loss of the scientific rigour that is required for its evaluation. Having briefly outlined the case against, we will now make the case in favour of the diagnostic process.

Why classify? The case for

Probably the most important reason for attempting to describe and categorize psychopathology is that abnormal mental states cause considerable suffering and disability. As well as causing morbidity, abnormal mental states also lead to increased mortality, which is partly, but not solely, due to the high rates of suicide among those who experience them. In the past little could be done to treat such distress, but this is now no longer the case. Drug treatment, in particular, is both powerful and effective in substantially reducing or even eliminating many symptoms. In addition, there are now several forms of psychotherapy (or 'talking treatment' methods) which have also been shown to be highly effective in alleviating the distress caused by psychopathology. In order to determine which treatment will be most effective it is necessary to *identify* the psychopathology and assign the individual to a *category* of mental disorder.

The individual's unique personal experience is certainly important in modifying both the presenting features as well as their response to treatment. Nonetheless, there is now a considerable body of research evidence which shows that certain diagnostic groups respond preferentially to certain types of treatment but not to others. For example, lithium carbonate is an effective mood stabilizer for individuals with bipolar disorder, but is of little benefit in the treatment of schizophrenia. Hence, it is necessary to assign individuals to a specific diagnostic group, which will then indicate what treatment is most appropriate. In addition, assigning an individual to a group with others who share similar psychopathological features in common allows predictions to be made about the future course and outcome.

Another reason for categorizing mental disorders is to address the needs of sufferers and plan services. If we fail to distinguish between different categories of mental disorder, or between mental disorder and health, we also fail to separate the different needs of someone with psychotic symptoms from someone who has an anxiety state.

The treatments currently available for these two disorders are quite different. It is also important for those planning services, for example, day care facilities, to know whether they have to provide places for 50, 200 or 1,000 individuals.

Even if it is agreed that the case has been made for categorizing psycho-pathology, there remain a number of further issues. These relate to i) problems with the terminology, ii) the disease concept when applied to mental disorders and iii) the case for replacing current diagnostic systems with a dimensional approach.

Problems of terminology

Mental experiences can be described verbally, and expressed in writing, or artwork such as painting. Consequently such experiences require the ability to communicate intimate thoughts and feelings which may be open to varied interpretation. Many everyday words have been used to describe psychopathology e.g. guilt, worry, tension, but their precise definition may become confused with their 'lay' meaning. Some have lost their meaning in translation from other languages. For example, many Anglo-American psychopathological terms have derived from the English translations of the writings of German and French phenomenologists and psychiatrists (Jaspers 1963, Esquirol 1833). In addition, some of the special terms used in psychiatry have been taken over into ordinary parlance, so that their meaning has been altered (e.g. the use of the term 'schizophrenic' to mean split personality).

Because psychiatrists have trained as doctors their response to the presence of psychopathology is to talk about 'illness' and 'disease'. However, there are considerable problems about the definition of disease or illness when applied to psychopathology. This problem is not unique to psychiatry. Other branches of medicine may have similar problems, but as we have outlined above, the criticism of applying the disease concept to those exhibiting psychopathology has been quite vociferous. Hence we will now review various definitions of 'disease' and 'illness' and indicate how these are problematic when applied to subjects exhibiting psychopathology.

Definitions of 'disease'

The most straightforward definition of disease was that proposed by Cohen (1960) who stated that a disease was a 'statistical deviation from the average'. While this definition is simple and objective, it is has the disadvantage that individuals, for example, with a very high IQ or who are very tall, are now defined as diseased.

According to Scadding (1967) a disorder is 'an excess or defect in some common characteristic by which they differ from the norm for their species in a biologically disadvantageous way'. Scadding allowed for the fact that 'disadvantage' may be only statistical rather than applied to each individual with a disorder. However the main problem with Scadding's definition is that the term 'biological disadvantage' now requires its own definition.

Kraupl Taylor (1971) gave the following definition: 'Disorder exists when there is a difference in the characteristic from the norm, and the difference either arouses therapeutic concern in the individual, or in society or both'. Although this definition emphasizes the personal or public concern about an illness and the need for treatment or prevention, this definition also allows political dissent to be included as a disorder. For example, in the Communist era in the Soviet Union, the term 'sluggish schizophrenia' was often applied to political dissidents as an excuse to incarcerate them (Tomov 1999).

Yet another definition of a mental disorder is that 'this exists where there is distress, disability and/or impaired reality testing' (Schofield 1966). In this definition the inclusion of 'impaired reality testing' will include individuals with psychotic symptoms, even if they are functioning well as having a disorder. However, distress and disability are not quantified and can occur in the absence of psychopathology.

Arguably, a more reasonable definition for a mental disorder is that of Kendell (1975). Kendell's definition is essentially the same as that of Scadding, but the author defines 'biological disadvantage' as requiring either the decline of fertility or reduction of the lifespan. Although this definition is more explicit than Scadding's, it is perhaps a little too much so. A number of disorders that clearly cause suffering and pain would not be included in this definition, for example, dental caries, but individuals who chose a celibate life style or those who are exclusively homosexual would be included.

The most recent and comprehensive definition of a mental disorder has been produced in an operational format (see chapter 3 for a more detailed description of what is meant by an operational definition) by Spitzer and Endicott (1978). In this definition the following criteria must be fulfilled for the condition to be considered a mental disorder.

The condition, in its fully developed or extreme form, occurs in all environments, (other than one especially created to compensate for the

---

Box 1.1 Definitions of disease

Statistical deviation from the average	Cohen (1960)
Biologically disadvantageous deviation from the norm	Scadding (1967)
Differences arouse therapeutic concern	Kraupl Taylor (1971)
Disorder exists where there is distress, disability and/or impaired reality testing	Schofield (1966)
Biological disadvantage causes decline in fertility or shortened life span	Kendell (1975)
Operational definition: condition associated with distress, disability or disadvantage	Spitzer and Endicott (1975)
Clinically recognized set of symptoms or behaviour associated with distress and/or interference with personal functions	World Health Organization (1992)

---

condition), is directly associated with:

A1 Distress acknowledged by the individual or manifest.

A2 Disability (some impairment and functioning in wide range of activities) or

A3 Disadvantage, other than resulting from A1/A2 – certain forms of disadvantage to the individual in interacting with aspects of the physical or social environment because of an identifiable psychological or social factor.

B The controlling variables tend to be attributed largely within the organism (either for initiating or maintaining factors). Except if giving information or 'non-technical' interventions are successful in reversing the condition.

C The condition is not included as a disorder if the associated distress, disability or other disadvantage is the apparently necessary price for attaining some positive goal.

This definition detaches distress from disability, which is helpful when considering the wider range of mental disorders that are considered to be treatable, or the focus for research interest. The definition also excludes those who have chosen a celibate life style. However, there remain a number of problems with this definition, including what is meant by 'non-technical' interventions etc.

An acceptable 'working' definition for a mental disorder is that included in the International Classification of Diseases tenth edition (ICD-10) (World Health Organization 1992). The ICD-10 states that

> Disorder is not an exact term but is used here to imply the existence of a clinically recognisable set of symptoms or behaviour associated in most cases with distress and with interference with personal functions. Social deviants or conflict alone, without personal dysfunction should not be included in mental disorder as defined here. This definition will cause some difficulties with those socially deviant individuals who are said to have a psychopathic personality disorder since such individuals would not be included in the ICD-10 definition of mental disorder. However the definition does include the need for a 'clinically recognisable set of symptoms or behaviour'. While this definition is practical, applicable, generally acceptable and has face validity, nonetheless it brings us full circle back to the importance of accurately measuring the signs and symptoms of mental disorder.

Dimensions and categories

So far, we have discussed the categorical approaches to the measurement of psychopathology which clinicians employ in order to diagnose and treat mental disorders. We have alluded to some of the problems and criticisms of this approach, which are mainly to do with the reliability and validity of diagnosis. We will discuss these in more detail in chapters 3 and 4. Some researchers have proposed that using a dimensional approach to measure psychopathology would have greater validity (Persons 1986, Bentall *et al.* 1990, Costello 1992). We will examine some of their reasoning by returning to our earlier example of 'worrying'.

It is clear that worrying is a universal human experience, which only becomes pathological when severe and prolonged. Thus worrying can be considered as a dimension, ranging from mild and self-limiting to pervasive and severe. The detailed clinical enquiry we described above enables the clinician or researcher to elicit how much the respondent has worried. It is then possible to place the individual respondent's experience on the dimension of worry. A severity/duration cut-off point determines whether the respondent's worrying is pathological or not. Thus the 'worry dimension' is converted into a dichotomy; pathological/not pathological. Similarly, adding together the number, type and severity of symptoms and signs into syndromes can also be considered to produce a severity dimension of psychopathology. Again, where the individual respondent's sign/symptom profile lies on this dimension determines whether they are considered 'cases' of mental disorder (Wing *et al.* 1981). Imposing such cutoffs on dimensions in this way has been considered arbitrary and possibly spurious. A good case can be made for allocating more research time to the study of symptoms (Costello 1992) although others have suggested that adopting a dimensional approach has limitations (Mojtabai and Rieder 1998). We will return to this discussion in more detail in chapter 10.

In chapter 2, we will describe the signs and symptoms that are considered to be psychopathological.

Describing Symptoms and Signs

Diagnostic building blocks

The description of signs and symptoms is the first stage in the measurement of psychopathology. Signs and symptoms can be regarded as the basic building blocks from which diagnostic categories are constructed. Also, they often provide the basis for items used in constructing continuous measures such as clinical rating scales (see chapters 1, 7 and 10). Traditionally, most emphasis has been on symptoms, the things of which patients complain, and psychiatry has sometimes been described as 'neurology without physical signs' (Miller 1961). This is not strictly true, because important parts of a mental state examination include direct observations of, for example, the individual's behaviour, appearance and form of speech (signs). That said, most research, dating back to the introduction of structured or semi-structured interviews (Wing *et al.* 1974) (see also chapter 5) shows that the rating of symptoms tends to more reliable than the rating of signs.

In this chapter we will attempt to give a concise overview of the mental state examination and the main symptoms and signs encountered in those with mental disorders. There are of course entire classic texts (e.g. Schneider 1959, Jaspers 1963, Fish 1974) devoted to this topic, as well as some excellent and perhaps more accessible recent counterparts (e.g. Sims 1988). In addition to discussing the main types of signs and symptoms found in adults (including the elderly), we will also consider in this chapter the different presentations of psychopathology found in children and adolescents, as well as the abnormalities or delay of normal development that may be associated with psychopathology.

This chapter is therefore principally about descriptive *psychopathology*, a term which is often used as if it were synonymous with *phenomenology*, a term which has entered psychiatry and psychology largely due to the influence of Jaspers (1963). However, as we have already mentioned in chapter one, it is worth noting that in the strict sense in which it was originally used, phenomenology means not just the description of symptoms and the mental state, but also the empathic understanding of how such states arrive. In other words, the person carrying out the mental state examination tries to put his or herself in the place of the subject and tries to work out the *meaningful connections* between experiences, thoughts and feelings. Jaspers also believed that one of the key features of psychotic symptoms that differentiate them from other sorts of symptoms is that they are essentially *non-understandable*. However, in this chapter we will not attempt to describe psychopathology in a strictly phenomenological way. Rather we will stick with simple descriptions and cover most of the main symptoms that provide the components of modern diagnostic criteria, such as those contained in the Diagnostic and Statistical Manual fourth edition (DSMIV) (American Psychiatric Association 1994), and the International Classification of Diseases tenth edition (ICD-10) (World Health Organization 1993) (see also chapter 3).

The mental state

Conventionally an individual's mental state is described under a number of separate headings. This might at first seem arbitrary and restrictive but it follows the precedent of both general medicine, with its division of the body into 'systems' (e.g. cardiovascular, respiratory, central nervous) and of traditional psychology, which describes mental life according to various processes (e.g. emotion, cognition). Of course such divisions are artificial, but they serve the same purpose as in medicine and psychology, that of facilitating observation and description.

Inevitably technical terms need to be used in describing mental states and indeed technical terms are employed throughout the two major international diagnostic systems (currently, ICD10 [WHO 1992], and DSMIV [APA 1998]). However it is better to be generally wary of technical terms and to avoid altogether those that one is not prepared to define in plain English. When writing clinical or research notes about mental states, it is often most valuable to give a jargon free description of the individual's experiences in every day terms. For example, 'Mr. X was convinced he was the wickedest man in the world and heard the voice of God telling him that he deserved to be severely punished' is altogether more informative and almost as succinct as 'Mr X suffered from delusions of guilt and auditory hallucinations'.

Appearance and behaviour

This is the part of the mental health examination that depends most on the direct observations made by the examiner, rather than the subject's self-report. As such it should be easy, but as we have noted it tends to be the poorest part of an interview in achieving inter-rater agreement (Wing et al. 1974). It helps to try and give a lifelike description of the individual in a few sentences and concentrate on the following characteristics:

Manner (in relation to the interview and interviewer)

Is the subject hostile, aggressive or amiable and helpful? How does the subject respond to the interviewer? Are they willing to talk about their feelings, thoughts etc., or reluctant to do so? Is the subject over-familiar or inappropriately seductive?

Dress and self-care

Is the subject tidy and well-groomed, or unkempt with poor hygiene?

Posture and movement

Is the subject relaxed or tense and restless, slowed up, overactive? Are there any abnormal movements, gestures or grimaces?

Appropriateness

Does the subject seem to be in touch with what is going on around him or does he appear perplexed, puzzled or disorientated? Are there any bizarre features in this behaviour, for example appearing to be listening or responding to auditory hallucinations?

Facial appearance

Does the subject look frightened or anxious, happy or smiling, or suspicious? People who are depressed may also be 'putting on a brave face', i.e. attempting to smile or show an animated expression. However, observation shows that the facial expression is only coming from the bottom half of the face, while the eyes show the underlying despair. This is termed *depressive facies*.

Abnormalities of movement and behaviour

So-called 'psychomotor' abnormalities are very common even in mildly abnormal mental states, but are frequently over looked. The most common abnormality is *restlessness*, which can occur in the context of anxiety or, in childhood, as a persistent feature in attention deficit hyperactivity disorder (ADHD). The main difference between restlessness or anxiety and ADHD is that the anxious subject appears fearful and distressed, whereas typically the individual with ADHD does not. Other motor accompaniments of anxiety include *tremor* at rest. This is typically described as a *fine tremor* and can be examined by asking the subject to stretch out their arms in front of them with their fingers spread and palms downward. It is important to note that many of the drugs used to treat mental disorders also cause a tremor, so it is also necessary to enquire about this as a possible cause.

In addition, there are some physical illnesses where tremor occurs as part of the clinical picture. However, the metabolic disorder that most commonly has to be differentiated from restlessness and tremor caused by chronic anxiety, is that caused by an overactive thyroid gland (thyrotoxicocosis), where a blood test will show raised levels of thyroid hormones. In addition, thyrotoxicocosis is frequently associated with eye abnormalities and a swelling of the thyroid gland in the neck (goitre). A useful differentiation in more subtle cases is that the hands are usually cold and clammy in anxiety, but feel warm in thyrotoxicocosis. In contrast, the anxious individual shows other obvious features of over arousal including *sweating* and *pallor*. The extreme of over-arousal is seen in someone who is experiencing a panic attack; who in addition to looking terrified, and being restless, may also over-breathe, complain of pins and needles in the hands, and even show muscular spasms of hands and forearms known as *tetany*.

Agitation is one of those difficult terms to define, because in the context of describing psychopathology it has a technical meaning which is slightly different from everyday usage. Agitation classically occurs in the context of severe depression and in addition to restlessness, the agitated individual shows repetitive motor activity such as wringing of hands, rocking, or pacing up and down, accompanied by the facial appearance of mental anguish. Alternatively, severe depression may be accompanied by *retardation*, in which the individual shows slowing of movements and delayed responses. The over activity seen in mania can be regarded as the polar opposite to depression, whereby the individual is not just restless, but constantly 'on the go'. Unlike the restlessness seen in agitated depression, someone with mania is subjectively full of energy and tries to direct this to what seem to them to be sensible goals, even if these do not seem to be sensible to the detached observer. One example is that of a woman who stayed up all night for several nights in a row, repeatedly cleaning her house from top to bottom.

Catatonic symptoms and signs

These days, catatonic symptoms and signs are rare, but were a lot more common before the time of effective treatment for psychosis. These very striking behaviours are occasionally seen in individuals in the acute stage of psychotic illnesses before there has been a response to treatment. Catatonic symptoms and signs include a number of different types of abnormal behaviours and movements. These are *mannerisms, stereotypies, waxy flexibility, catalepsy, catatonic excitement and stupor. Mannerisms* are embellishments or adornments of normal movements, which many of us exhibit to some extent. Consequently some mannerisms can be regarded as within the normal range. However, individuals with psychotic disorders may show bizarre mannerisms that are usually associated with a delusional explanation. For example, a young woman walked in a slightly stooped way with her right arm held behind her back and up between her shoulder blade. Her explanation for walking this way was that she had been 'posed by God'. Another young man made a clicking, coughing noise each time he spoke accompanied by a shaking of his head. He explained that this was to 'clear the evil out of my throat'.

Stereotypies are repetitive movements that look deliberate but which are in fact purposeless, for example saluting or arm flapping.

In the classic catatonic state, the individual has an abnormality of muscle tone that is termed *waxy flexibility*. This refers to feeling of 'moving through wax' that an examiner experiences when attempting to passively move the catatonic subject's arm at the elbow.

Maintaining abnormal or uncomfortable postures for long periods (even those in which the individual has been placed by others) is termed *catalepsy*. One of the most striking examples of catalepsy is the *'psychological pillow'* which fortunately is rarely seen, when the subject lies for long periods on a bed with their head slightly raised off the real pillow.

In *catatonic excitement* there is extreme and disruptive overactivity, whereas in *catatonic stupor* the opposite occurs. The person experiencing *catatonic stupor* lies motionless and appears to be awake in that the eyes are usually open or can be opened, and will follow the observer around the room. Nevertheless, the individual is unresponsive to conversation or even painful stimuli. Typically, there is also incontinence of urine and faeces.

Although catatonic signs have been considered as essentially a component of schizophrenia, they actually usually occur in the context of other disorders, particular affective illness. Stupor in particular can be seen as an extreme form of retardation. Catatonic signs and symptoms also occur in the context of drug induce states and organic brain syndromes.

Abnormalities of speech

When considering an individual's speech it is important to distinguish between the form and content of their conversation. In order to understand the difference between *form* and *content*, consider this book. For example, the *form* of this volume is that it is a small book printed in English. On the other hand, its *content* is the measurement of psychopathology. Therefore, the *form* of speech comprises its structure, grammar and syntax as well as its flow, i.e. the speed of utterance, while the content refers to the topic of the conversation. In the case of someone expressing delusional beliefs, the speech content may also show abnormalities (these are discussed later in this chapter). The important observations are whether the subject is able to give a coherent account or one that is difficult to understand. For example, are there frequent changes of topic or does one topic follow logically on from the next? Is there a long delay before a question is answered or is the speech so rapid that it comes out 'under pressure'. In order to decide whether there is a disorder of speech it is useful to write down what the person is saying, verbatim.

Abnormalities of the form of speech

How best to describe the abnormalities of speech found in psychotic disorders has provoked considerable debate. Even the traditional term, *formal thought disorder* has been severely criticized on the grounds that it is strictly the subject's speech that has been observed, and speech is only indirectly related to the expression of thoughts. That said, subjects who show abnormalities of speech frequently show similar abnormalities in their written communications, suggesting that there is some disorder in the way thinking is structured. The simpler scheme is simple to consider formal speech (or thought) disorders under the headings of positive, negative and pressures of speech.

Positive formal speech disorder

As its most basic, abnormal speech is that which makes communication difficult because of lack of logical or understandable organization. We can all be accused of showing this sign at times, and almost anyone who has had the unedifying experience of having an extended piece of conversation written down verbatim will realize that grammatical errors, pauses, 'hums', 'arhs' and unfinished sentences are a universal affliction. Nevertheless, most people maintain a sufficient degree of form to communicate what they mean to say, most of the time. The key feature about positive formal thought disorder is that this no longer pertains. The subject may have fluent speech but may use words in a bizarre or idiosyncratic way or invent new ones (*neologisms*). There is also what Bleuler (1950) originally described as '*loosening of association*' when each phrase or fragment of speech is poorly connected with the phrase or fragment that goes before and after. The theme of the speech may become '*derailed*', that is figuratively it appears to be going down one track before suddenly switching to another and then yet another. In its most severe form, speech becomes totally '*incoherent*'. This is traditionally described as a '*word salad*', where it is as if the words have been merely thrown together and tossed into a jumble.

Negative formal speech disorder

Typically here the individual shows *paucity of thought* and may show frequent *thought blocking*. This is again an exaggerated form of a phenomenon with which most people are familiar in stressful circumstances. Actors know it as 'drying', that is, suddenly forgetting the lines during a performance. In everyday life, most people will have had the experience of occasionally forgetting what they were about to say. In a schizophrenic illness characterized by negative formal speech disorder this phenomenon can become frequent and intense, and is often accompanied by a delusional explanation (see also *thought withdrawal*, later in this chapter).

Poverty of speech or thought can also occur in schizophrenic illnesses. This relates to the paucity of verbal utterances, despite the individual appearing to be cooperating with the discussion: limited responses such as 'yes' or 'no' are given to questions that require a more detailed reply. Similarly, there is *poverty of content of speech* when the subject replies to a question with several sentences, but manages to convey very little information. Again if the observer thinks that either poverty of speech or poverty of content of speech is present, it is helpful to write down verbatim what the subject says. This verbatim account can be examined later, when it usually becomes apparent that one or other of these abnormalities of speech is present.

Pressure of speech

Pressure or 'push' of speech occurs when the subject is far more talkative than usual or feels a pressure to continue talking. In its more severe forms the speech continues in an unstoppable flow which the listener cannot interrupt, and which does not cease even when it becomes obvious that the listener is no longer paying attention. It is usually associated with *flight of ideas*, which is characterized by a rapid stream of thought connected by puns, rhymes and plays on words, usually of a rudimentary form known as 'clang association'. Such speech patterns classically occur in mania and, in contrast with loosening of associations found in schizophrenic formal thought disorder, it is usually possible to follow the train of thought despite the inherent eccentricities. For example a woman was asked to explain the proverb 'a stitch in time saves nine'. She replied 'it's when you've got a cut and it needs a stitch. A stitch in time saves nine. Nine lives. Nine lives like a cat. I've got a little black cat actually'.

Some individuals show a milder form of pressured speech in which the output is excessive, and this is sometime referred to as *prolixity*. This may be accompanied by *circumstantiality* when the subject insists on giving a blow by blow account in reply to every question, insisting on going into meticulous detail and taking a long time coming to the point. Circumstantiality in the absence of pressured speech is most commonly associated with obsessional personality traits rather than with manic states. However, circumstantiality can also occur as part of normal speech patterns. Senior professors, as well as those with learning disability, may have circumstantial speech!

Abnormalities of mood

In describing an individual's mood, it is important to note the subjective report and decide whether it is in keeping with the appearance and behaviour. If there is a complaint of low mood or depression it is important to know the subject's outlook for the future and whether there are any associated suicidal ideas or plans. A morbid degree of elation may be more difficult to judge from the individual's subjective account alone. However, some will admit to feeling 'too high' or 'too cheerful to be normal'; in addition to classical elation a 'high' mood may be associated with irritability or hostility.

Depression

Periods of sadness or low mood are part of everyday experience and, fortunately, are usually self-limiting. The symptom of depression, like pain, is highly ubiquitous. It can therefore become a real challenge to decide at what stage 'normal' depression becomes a symptom of clinical significance. The rough and ready answer, as with any symptom, is when it causes impairment. However, it is possible to go somewhat further than this and, as with pain, there is the standard set of questions than can be asked to grade severity (see chapter 5 for more details about severity rating in depresson). Thus, does depression persist all the time or does it come and go? Is it worse at any particular time? Typically in *'endogenous'* depression, the mood is lowest in the mornings. However, for many people with severe depression this is not the case, and, particularly when depression is mixed with anxiety, patients describe feeling worse towards the end of the day.

Does anything make the depression worse (e.g. being reminded of the loss of a love one)? Does anything make it better? Typically, in the most severe cases of depression, the person becomes unresponsive to social cues and cannot be distracted from their feelings of despair.

What does the depression make the person want to do? Frequently it will make them want to cry, although many subjects with severe depression say that they have 'gone beyond' crying. More worryingly, depression is frequently associated with thoughts of suicide, suicidal plans and acts. All these need to be asked about explicitly, and usually in that order. Such ideas are nearly always associated with self-depreciation, self-criticism and often with feelings of guilt and worthlessness.

Anhedonia, or inability to obtain enjoyment, is a common accompaniment of depression, and may sometimes be the presenting symptom in a depressive disorder, even in the absence of the subjective complaint of low mood. Loss of appetite for food can be seen as a particular form of anhedonia, and most subjects who complain of diminished appetite and weight loss in depression, describe a loss of interest in food rather than an overt aversion to eating. Some subjects show the reverse of typical appetite loss and instead gain weight, which they may ascribe to 'comfort eating'. This is sometime seen in mixed anxiety and depression, but it also occurs in individuals with seasonal exacerbation of recurrent depression during winter months (seasonal affective disorder or SAD). Also associated with a seasonal pattern of depression is excessive sleeping or *hypersomnia,* which suggests parallels with states of hibernation in some animals.

Anxiety

Abnormal mood states predominated by anxiety can occur in a non-specific way as in *generalized anxiety disorder* or in specific circumstances, so called *phobic anxiety.* Probably the most common provoking agent or cues of phobic anxiety are social situations, followed by *agoraphobia* (literally 'fear of the marketplace') where anxiety is provoked by public places such as shops or supermarkets or travelling on public transport. Overt panic attacks are rare in *social phobia,* but fear of having such an attack or of 'doing something stupid' may be intense, as is the embarrassment of showing the symptoms of autonomic arousal such as sweating, mentioned earlier.

By contrast in agoraphobia, *panic attacks* are common and an important and frightening subjective symptom is *angor animi*, or a feeling of impending doom. In severe anxiety states, *depersonalization* can become a worrisome feature. Here the individual has the intense feeling that they are not any longer a person and experience the associated phenomenon of *derealization*, when they are feel detached from the world or that they are not living in a real world. Such feelings often come on in the midst of a panic attack. Fleeting feelings of depersonalization or derealization come particularly at a time of stress, and are probably experienced by most people – particularly so by introspective individuals. In anxiety states, depersonalization and derealization are usually short lived, lasting minutes or at most hours. Depersonalization lasting longer than this is rare, and if it does occur, is usually seen in the context of acute psychotic disorders.

Mania and hypomania

Manic states are usually associated with elevated or 'high' mood when the subject feels very happy, confident, full of ideas and plans. In classic elation, the high mood of the subject is described as infectious and is akin, in exaggerated form, to the consistent jollity of the hyperthymic individual who enjoys being the 'life and soul of the party'. Alternatively the manic subject may be very irritable or angry, mainly because no one else can keep up with his/her activities and plans. This is more likely to occur in a persistent manic state or in individuals who have had multiple episodes of mania. Associated with the excessive over activity is an exaggerated sense of self worth, rapid speech and thinking (see above), feckless or inappropriate behaviour which is out of keeping with the way the person usually acts, overspending and sometimes even sexual indiscretions. The latter can cause both financial problems and/or considerable embarrassment when the subject is no longer manic. The manic person has limited sleep, usually only a few hours each night, but this gives them more time for their schemes and plans, so there are no subjective complaints about the insomnia. Rather it is other people who complain about the excess activity especially if this takes place throughout the night. For example one man decided to cut his lawn at 4 am – his neighbours were not pleased at their sleep being disturbed by the sound of his lawn mower.

In severe manic states, the individual loses touch with reality and may develop delusions and/or hallucinations. These are usually *mood congruent* i.e. related to grandiose abilities or identity (see later in this chapter). Also, overactivity and lack of sleep can lead to profound exhaustion. People with this severity of manic symptoms are usually admitted to hospital fairly rapidly, as their overactive behaviour usually draws the attention of the police or other authorities.

Content of thought

It is important here to note the person's current concerns, worries, pre-occupations and fears. These may be about self or others and may relate to present circumstances only or include past concerns. As discussed in chapter 1, most abnormal thought content in common psychiatric disorders is on a continuum with 'normal' worries, so that it is important to judge the extent to which thought content is constant and troublesome and whether the person can readily turn their mind to other things.

Abnormal beliefs and ideas

The most striking and clear-cut abnormal beliefs are termed *delusions*. To be classified as a delusion an abnormal beliefs must fulfil three criteria. First, it must clearly be false, second, it must be relatively fixed, unshakeable, and not amenable to reason, and third, it must be out of keeping with the individual's cultural, education or religious background. This third component requires particular careful consideration. This is because beliefs that are widely accepted within one particular cultural, religious or ethic group may seem strange, unacceptable or even bizarre to another. Religious beliefs provide the most striking examples, throwing out differences even between different branches of the same faith. Thus, members of a fundamental Christian church who have beliefs in keeping with a literal interpretation of New Testament scriptures, are likely to hold different views about supernatural phenomenon to someone who has been raised broadly as a Christian, but who has no current religious affiliation. Sensitivity to the person's background becomes even more important in societies where there has been a recent admixture of diverse ethic groups.

Types of delusions

One way of classifying delusions is as those that concern (a) the outside world (b) the self and (c) outside influences on the self.

Delusions concerning the outside world

Delusions of persecution are by far the commonest variety. In one fairly typical study of subjects suffering from schizophrenia, persecutory delusions were reported by over 70% (Farmer *et al.* 1983). Delusions of persecution range from the vague ('someone is out to get me') to the very specific (e.g. 'X is trying to kill me by poisoning my food'). Because these are the commonest form of delusion and the most frequently described abnormal beliefs in *paranoid states*, the term 'paranoid delusion' and delusion of persecution are sometimes used interchangeably. It has been argued by some writers that this is both imprecise and tautological, because paranoid literally means 'beside the mind' or deluded!

The other very common type of delusion that can occur in any form of paranoid disorder is a *delusion of reference*. A less severe non-delusional form of this experience is termed *ideas of reference,* which may be understandable. For example, most people placed in an unfamiliar or anxiety-provoking situation are capable of feeling acutely self-conscious and perhaps wondering whether a word exchanged between two strangers on the other side of the room might somehow be a remark about them. This is sometimes call a *simple idea of reference* (Wing *et al.* 1974). Usually it is shrugged off without further concern, but some individuals with non-psychotic depression or severe anxiety disorders report persistent states of acute self-consciousness where simple ideas of reference occur fairly frequently.

Delusions of reference differ from normal experience in a more clear cut way, in that the person has an unshakeable belief that people are talking about them behind their back and that this may be in the context of a scheme or plot to harm them (thus delusions of persecution and of reference frequently coexist). Delusions of self-reference may become even more outlandish with the person describing messages about themselves or signals that are meant to convey a message or meaning being planted in the newspaper, the radio or the television. For example a young man watching a television news programme noticed that the newsreader appeared to grimace at one point and realized that this was the message that he, the viewer, was being pursued by MI5.

Delusions concerning the self

By far the commonest delusion in this category is that of *grandiosity*. These may consist of a markedly inflated sense of self-importance such that the individual believes that they have assumed the identity of a person or being who is rich, famous, or divine, or that they have special powers or abilities. Delusions of *grandiose identity* need to be interpreted, as with any other abnormal belief, against the subject's particular background. While claims of divinity usually indicate that the claimant is deluded, subcultural influences may be difficult to disentangle. Thus for example a unsophisticated young woman from a rural part of Sri Lanka 'discovered' that she had become a Buddha and for sometime was encouraged in this belief by her family and neighbours, until her behaviour became overtly psychotic in other ways. On the other hand some people with more modest assertions about acquired identity are obviously delusional, such as a man in his thirties of limited educational attainments who stated that on his first admission to hospital he had fared so well that he had been created a professor of psychiatry!

Delusions of grandiose ability encompass special powers or talent. Once again these range from the outlandish and supernatural through to the physically possible, and need to be interpreted against the person's background. Hence a claim of miraculous powers of healing needs to be interpreted cautiously, if the individual belongs to a religious denomination where this will not be out of place. On the other hand, a young man who said that he had acquired mathematical ability equivalent to Einstein, despite having no formal educational qualifications, was certainly deluded. Grandiosity is most typically found in manic states, but can occur in schizophrenia and other paranoid states when it may coexist with delusion of persecution and self-reference.

Self-depreciation, which in its extreme form amounts to *delusion of worthlessness,* can be seen as the opposite and is most often found in severe depressive disorder. *Delusions of guilt* may be simple and vague ('I'm a bad person') or more take on a more complicated and overtly bizarre form, such as a middle aged man who believes that he was personally responsible for the deaths or injuries of British soldiers involved in the 1991 Gulf war. Less common are delusions of bodily change. These can sometimes be the only abnormality in the mental state. For example, in so-called *monosymptomatic delusional syndromes,* an individual may be convinced that some part of their appearance such as their nose or part of their body is misshaped, despite any real objective evidence to support to this. This syndrome is sometimes called *dysmorphophobia,* but this is really an inappropriate term, since it means fear of being misshapen. In severe depressive states *nihilistic delusions* may occur. These consist of beliefs that a part of the body has

---

Box 2.1 Assessment of the mental state

Appearance and behaviour
Abnormalities of speech
Abnormalities of mood
Thought content
Abnormalities of perception (delusions and hallucinations)
Abnormalities of cognition

---

disappeared or become damaged (for example 'my brain has rotted away' or 'my innards have been completely eaten by maggots'). Another delusion that is sometime seen in severe depression (and again might be regarded as the opposite of manic grandiosity) concerns *poverty*: the person believes that they have become financially ruined or that all their possession have been taken away.

Delusions concerning outside influences on the self

Two groups of delusions have sometimes been classified as indicating 'ego boundary' problems when the individual has difficulties distinguishing between themselves and the outside world. These consist of *delusions of passivity* and *thought interference*.

The subject experiencing *delusions of passivity* believes that they are under the control of some force, power or agency, other than themselves. This results in their actions being controlled (*'made' actions*), and the description that they are being moved about like a puppet on a string. Sometimes the subject will be able to elaborate, on how this has been effected. For example, a young woman believed that her actions were being controlled by the pop singer David Bowie, by means of a radio transmission device that he has implanted into her head. Alternatively, the individual may simply experience 'made' impulses without acting upon them. For example, a young man described having the repeated impulse to throw himself onto railway lines in front of oncoming trains, and describe this as being imposed upon him by the spirit of his now deceased great uncle. Some subjects may also describe *'made' sensations* which are most commonly tactile, and less frequently, imposed or *'made' emotions* may be described.

Thought interference can take a variety of forms. In *thought withdrawal*, there is the belief that the thoughts have suddenly disappeared out of the individual's head so that no thoughts are left behind. This may sometimes be given as an explanation for the phenomenon of thought blocking described earlier. *Thought insertion* describes the opposite phenomenon, in which thoughts are put into the person's head by some outside agency. These experiences are usually upsetting or disturbing. *Thought broadcasting* is the belief that one's thoughts can actually be heard by others. For example, a young woman who lived in a therapeutic hostel explained that she never said anything in-group meetings because other members could already hear her thoughts.

Primary delusions

Delusions arising 'out of the blue', and not preceded by any other overt symptoms, are termed *primary delusions*. Three main types occur. *Primary delusional ideas* are the most straightforward in that they involve the sudden occurrence of a fully formed belief, which may be described as coming to the individual like a revelation. These may have a grandiose quality ('I have suddenly come to realize that I am the Messiah') or a persecutory content ('Somehow the thought came to me that the IRA were out to kill me'). *Delusional mood* is a comparatively rare form of primary delusion that tends to occur at the beginning of psychotic illnesses with acute onset and may be associated with *perplexity* and or *depersonalization* (see below). The subject experiences a state lasting for days when there is an overwhelming feeling that something strange is happening which in some way is centred on them. Out of this rather amorphous state, delusions of reference and persecution then begin to crystallize.

Delusional perception describes the phenomenon of a delusional interpretation being suddenly placed, in a non-understandable way, on an everyday perception. There is what Schneider (1959) described as a 'two-membered' quality. For example a young man went into a church one day and noticed the smell of fresh paint (real perception). Immediately he knew that this was a sign that he was the victim of a plot involving his father, the church and the Boys Brigade (delusional interpretation). Perceptual theorists of the gestalt school have criticized Schneider's description, pointing out that all of the evidence suggests that when we perceive something, we perceive its totality and perceptions cannot therefore be broken down into components. This criticism is somewhat misplaced, however, since the point that Schneider was making was that the perception as such is perfectly commonplace but is believed by the subject to be a sign or a signal of something that is quite definitely out of the ordinary.

Obsessional thoughts and compulsive behaviour

Obsessions are repeated intrusive thoughts that the subject recognizes as their own, as irrational or unwanted and typically tries to resist. Resistance is usually associated with increased anxiety or mental discomfort and although it is sometimes described as a sine qua non, a proportion of individuals with chronic obsessive compulsive disorder appear to give up resisting and do not show this feature at all. It is worth noting that 'obsession' is a good example of a word that has an everyday general meaning that is somewhat different from the technical meaning used in connection with the descriptive psychopathology. Nevertheless, most people have experienced an obsession in the technical sense, for example a tune that goes round and round in one's head and which one cannot get rid of, or the strangely disturbing 'what if' thought that one might suddenly blurt out a profanity during some solemn occasion such a church service. Frequently, the content of obsessions are to do with ideas that have a magical or ritual-like quality, for example, thinking everything in multiples of threes or some other 'magic number'. Obsessions tend to be associated with *compulsions to* carry out certain repeated acts which, again, are regarded as irrational and tend to be resisted. Compulsions often follow the theme of cleansing or decontamination. Thus, a common obsession is of being unclean or contaminated by dirt, germs or bodily fluids, and this leads on to hand washing rituals. Frequently, the washing ritual has to be carried out in a particular way, or must be completed a specific number of times. Another common obsession is the feeling of 'incompleteness', that is, something that has not but should have been carried out. This again is an exaggerated form of everyday thoughts that most people have had ('did I lock the door?', 'did I turn the taps off?') In obsessive compulsive disorder, or sometimes in depressive state complicated by obsessions, obsessional doubts become exaggerated and intrusive and can lead to checking rituals where the taps, locks or the light switches have to be checked repeatedly, and again this may be in accordance with some 'magic' number.

Abnormal perceptions

Hallucinations are the commonest form of abnormal perception to occur in psychiatric disorder and can be defined as perceptions without stimuli. This is in contrast to *illusions* that consist of distorted or misinterpreted perceptions of stimuli that exist in reality. Illusions can occur at any time when information about the environment is ambiguous or misleading. This includes completely normal state, (e.g. walking home after dark in a poorly lit street when the imagination can play tricks on one) or in morbid states, most typically in toxic confusional disorders, such as delirium tremens, when frequent and frightening illusions dominate the clinical picture.

In psychological disorders not associated with confusion or dementia, *auditory hallucinations* represent the most common modality. *Elementary* hallucinations consist of noises or indistinct voices, or whispers where words cannot be made out. The commonest forms of distinct hallucinations in the form of voices usually have a derogatory or persecutory nature, usually addressing the subject in the second person. Continuous hallucinations with voices speaking in sentences are commonest in schizophrenia but can occur in affective disorders, either during a manic or severely depressed phase. Sometimes in mania, voices are in keeping with the subject's elated mood state and confirm their belief about their elevated status. In some individuals, usually those with chronic disorders with persistent hallucinations, the tone and content of the voices are neutral or even supportive.

It is important to note that people experiencing auditory hallucinations will usually describe hearing them through their ears, and will reply 'yes' to the question 'is the voice loud and clear like me talking to you now?' However, some people describe the voices as coming from 'inside my head'. There has been much debate as to whether these experiences occurring in 'subjective space' rather than definitely arising outside of the head should be described as *pseudo-hallucinations*, or whether the term should be reserved for hallucination like experiences, consisting of vivid, clear mental images that are to some extent under voluntary control (Mullen 1997).

Three types of auditory hallucinations are particularly characteristic of schizophrenia and were suggested by Schneider (1959) to be so-called first rank symptoms, any one of which, in the absence of 'brain disease' is diagnostic of schizophrenia (see also chapter 3 and Box 3.9). These are *third person auditory hallucinations, hallucinations providing a running commentary* and so called *thought echo.* (The other first rank symptoms listed by Schneider were the varieties of passivity phenomenon and thoughts interference mentioned earlier, together with delusional perception).

Third person auditory hallucinations consist of two or more voices, typically arguing or sometimes simply discussing the individual and referring to 'him' or 'her' or mentioning them by name. (This contrasts with the more usual derogatory voices, which refer to the subject in the second person as 'you'). *Running commentary* voices quite literally provide a description of the person's actions, as they take place. The term *thought echo* describes a phenomenon whereby at the same time as an individual is having a thought or immediately after, this is heard, spoken aloud, as a voice. This occasionally occurs in combination with the belief that thoughts are being broadcast. *Thought broadcast* refers to the idea that the subject's thoughts are passively diffusing out of his/her head, and are available to other people (Wing *et al.* 1974).

Hallucinations in other modalities

Olfactory hallucinations, that is abnormal perceptions involving smell or taste, can occur in a variety of disorders and are relatively non-specific. Olfactory hallucinations can occur in severe depressive states, and may coexist with nihilistic delusions (for example when the subject describes smelling their own rotting flesh). They can sometimes occur in schizophrenia, but are most characteristic of the so-called *aura*, that heralds the onset of a seizure in temporal lobe epilepsy.

Vivid *visual hallucinations* also tend to suggest a localized brain lesion and can occur along with focal epilepsy. However, drug-induced hallucinations are also an important cause and occur both with hallucinogens such as LSD and with some prescribed drugs such as the anticholinergic, benzhexol, or the antidepressant, venlafaxine. Drug withdrawal states can also cause visual hallucinations, the commonest and most well-known being those associated with withdrawal from alcohol (*delirium tremens*). Visual hallucinations can occur in schizophrenia and more rarely in mania, but tend to be neither vivid nor well formed.

Tactile hallucinations may result from drug-induced states. The classic example is cocaine intoxication, when the symptom of *formication* can occur, ie. the feeling that ants are crawling around under the skin. Tactile hallucinations also occur in schizophrenia (when as noted earlier the individuals may describe them as 'made' sensations) or less commonly in severe depression. These may be vague (e.g. 'tingling') or quite explicit (e.g. 'cold water running down the back of my neck'). As with olfactory hallucinations it is important to make sure that there is not a local physical explanation, such as a peripheral nerve lesion.

Occasionally subjects describe the experience of hallucinations occurring in multiple modalities e.g. hearing a voice and having a vision of the speaker of the voice at the same time. These have been described as *dissociative hallucinations* (Wing *et al.* 1974). Such hallucinations occasionally occur in the context of a schizophrenic illness, as well as in some people with temporal lobe epilepsy.

Abnormalities of cognition: general considerations

In the broad sense, *cognitive* simply means 'pertaining to thought', and there is now a whole branch of psychology, cognitive neuroscience, devoted to the study of cognition. This has lead to the realization that abnormalities of cognition may underlie the core features of a whole range of disorders including depression, schizophrenia and childhood autism. The term cognition also has a more restricted 'traditional' meaning in the context of mental state assessment, which has to do with abnormalities of intellect and memory, and it is in this more restricted sense that the term is used here.

It is impossible to make any judgement about abnormalities of intellect and memory without having some notion about premorbid levels of functioning. The best guide are schooling, age at leaving school, academic successes including exam passes, work record and career achievement. Clearly, none of these is a perfect indicator, but taken together provide a rough gauge of the level at which a subject might be expected to perform. In carrying out a general assessment is also important to note whether the subject is fully conscious and attentive or whether there is depression or a fluctuating level of consciousness. At the same time, it is important to observe whether the individual is generally orientated, whether they can provide a coherent account of their symptoms and whether there is an obvious difficulty in remembering places, names and dates.

Orientation

Disorientation is the hallmark of both confusional states and dementia. Disorientation may take place for time, that is, when the subject does not know date, day, or the approximate time of day without consulting a clock or watch. In disorientation for place the individual may not know where he is (i.e. the address) or even sometimes what type of place he is in. In the most extreme form, the subject may not even be able to choose correctly from a list of alternatives (e.g. 'is this a café, a church, a hospital or a railway station?'). Disorientated demented individuals may fail to recognize their close family members or spouses, but it is only in the most severe cases that the person will not be able to identify him or herself. There is also *age disorientation*, when the person can give his date of birth and even the current date correctly, but cannot correctly state his current age. This has been said to be one of the commonest cognitive abnormalities in chronic schizophrenia.

Attention and concentration

One of the hallmarks of acute confusional states is a gross disturbance of attention, with the subject showing a defective grasp of what is going on around them and, usually, a total inability to concentrate on anything for more than a few seconds. This is associated with a degree of unresponsiveness and a lowered conscious level, described as *clouding of consciousness*. Some individuals with acute psychosis also show profound attention problems, wear an expression of dazed puzzlement, and voice the belief that 'something strange' is happening. This state of *perplexity* may be associated with delusional mood (see above). Less acute attentional difficulties occur in dementia but it should be remembered that difficulty in concentration, often accompanied by problems in sustaining attention, is also a feature of severe depression. The average normal adult can usually repeat correctly a series of at least seven numbers and can provide a series of six in reverse order. This therefore is a useful clinical test as is saying the days of the week, or the months of the year, in reverse order.

Memory

A good indication of whether someone is having memory problems is their ability to recall recent developments of national or local news. Again, this ability needs to be interpreted against some assessment of the subject's premorbid level of functioning and the extent to which he or she normally reads the newspaper or watches the television news. If they say they follow the news rarely, other good alternatives are to ask about sport or recent 'events' on TV soap operas (but this presupposes that the interviewer also know about such things!). The average adult should be able to name the current Prime Minister (or President) and their two immediate predecessors. For someone who is a hospital inpatient, it is worth checking whether they can name the ward, the nurse in charge and what they had for their last meal.

Broadly speaking, two types of abnormalities may be found: the subject fails to give information or provides incorrect information. The latter, in its most blatant form, can amount to *confabulation* in which the person substitutes made up information for forgotten facts. For example, a man admitted to hospital for the investigation of his memory problems said that he had come into hospital for investigation of a broken leg and described how the doctors had carried out x-rays and discovered a broken thighbone. After giving this account he bade the interviewer good morning and walked normally out of the room.

Other abnormalities of registration and recall can be detected by asking the subject to repeat a name, address and the name of an object (for example, a flower or an animal) and testing whether these can be repeated immediately and again five minutes later. Individuals with registration or attentional difficulties may perform poorly at both, whereas those with other types of memory problem may specifically show poor delayed recall.

Language

Language abnormalities that disrupt the symbolic function of speech, such as *dysphasias or aphasias*, are associated with lesions in the dominant cerebral hemisphere. In most people this is the left hemisphere, but in about 3% of right-handed people, and in about 30–40% of those who are left-handed, the right hemisphere is dominant. The commonest abnormality is *nominal dyphasia*, and the commonest cause is an ischaemic lesion (i.e. a stroke). The person has word-finding difficulty that is most pronounced with words that are used with low frequency. For example, the person may be able to name parts of the body such as a 'hand' or 'finger', but may not be able to find the words for 'knuckle' or 'collarbone'.

Various complicated schemes have been devised to classify dysphasias, but for practical purposes they can be divided into *expressive* and *receptive* types. In general, expressive dysphasia occurs following an anterior lesion (the classic example being a lesion of Broca's area in the left frontal lobe) while receptive dysphasia results from a posterior lesion. Characteristically, expressive dysphasias are *non-fluent*; that is, the person produces little speech and has difficulty in coming out with what they want to say. By contrast the subject with receptive dysphasia shows *fluent* speech, but this is jumbled and difficult for the listener to understand. In severe form this is described as *jargon dysphasia* because the subject is, in effect, speaking an idiosyncratic language that only he or she can understand. In this respect there is a similarity with the severe varieties of formal thought disorder seen in schizophrenia, so that occasionally stroke patients whose main presenting symptom is language abnormality have been misdiagnosed as suffering from 'late onset schizophrenia'. In fact, marked language disorder is rare in schizophrenia presenting in middle age or beyond, so that a vascular or other focal lesion is always a more likely cause in this age group.

Visuospatial and constructional abnormalities

Visuospatial problems are not often complained about directly by the subject, but a clue as to their existence may be the onset of difficulties at work. Examples are a formerly successful heating engineer who found that he could no longer follow plans for installing new equipment, and a truck driver who began driving the wrong way around roundabouts. Such problems, as in both of these cases, usually result from parietal lobe lesions. Useful tests involve asking the person to draw a clock face, to write the numbers in the correct positions and to set the hands of the clock at a specific time. They can also be asked to copy a series of shapes of increasing difficulty, e.g. a triangle, a star, and a box drawn to show perspective in three dimensions. Impairment is usually greatest with right-sided (non dominant) hemisphere lesions when the outline and general orientation of the drawing is abnormal, whereas with left hemisphere lesions the problem is with internal details.

Dyscalculia

Acquired problems with handling numbers is again usually associated with parietal lobe lesions, and more severe when they occur in the dominant hemisphere. Testing involves asking the subject to perform simple mental arithmetic, e.g. subtractions, first without, and then with, carrying over (e.g. 45 take away 19). It is also customary to give the *serial 7's test*. The instructions for this test are as follows: 'Please take 7 from 100, then take 7 from the answer, and then take 7 from that answer, and continue until I ask you to stop'. You should write down the subject's series of answers, and note how long it takes. An adult of average intelligence should manage this task with no mistakes in under two minutes. However, in practice many people, even those who are not otherwise cognitively impaired, find the test difficult. You should make allowances for educational level, and the degree to which the subject is otherwise relaxed and attentive. This is not a 'pure' test of ability to calculate, as it also depends on attention and short-term memory. It is also important to test the subject's ability to do written calculations Again, start simply and assess the results against what you might expect given the subject's educational background.

Apraxia, agnosia and body image

Apraxia is the inability to carry out movements normally despite normal muscle power and normal gross coordination. It is usually associated with dominant parietotemporal lesions. A common symptom in late life is *dressing apraxia*, which in severe forms is obvious, but in milder cases can be tested for by asking the person to put on a coat or a dressing gown after an arm of the garment has been pulled inside out.

Acquired apraxia is often but not invariably associated with body image problems. These can be simply demonstrated by testing the person's ability to distinguish left and right (e.g. 'Please show me your left hand'). One should also test the person's ability to recognize parts of his body. The most common subtle abnormality is *finger agnosia*. This is tested for by asking the subject, 'please show me the little finger on your left hand', or 'please show me the thumb on your right hand'. A much more gross abnormality is *apropagnosia*, when the subject ignores or 'disowns' a limb or both limbs on one side of the body (nearly always the left). Most commonly this results from a stroke when the lesion is in the right (or non dominant) parietal lobe.

Descriptive psychopathology in children and adolescents

Angold (2000) points out that there have been major changes in the assessment of children over the past twenty-five years. These relate to the fairly recent recognition that children can be reliable informants about their own problems and difficulties. In addition, there have been similar developments in the assessment of psychopathology in children, as in adults. These include the introduction of operational diagnostic criteria for childhood disorders (operational definitions are described in chapter 3), as well as the structured interviews (these are discussed in chapter 5), and ratings scales (described in chapter 7) devised for their evaluation. These developments, that are further described in chapter 8, parallel those for adult disorders, and have led to the re-emergence of descriptive psychopathology in child and adolescent psychiatry (Angold 2000).

In addition to developmental disorders such as mental retardation, autistic spectrum, language and reading delays, the main categories of disorders in children and adolescents are emotional, and disruptive disorders (Scott 2000). Emotional disorders are largely the same as those in adults, namely anxiety, depression, phobias, and obsessive-compulsive disorder. Disruptive disorders are found more specifically in children, and include conduct and hyperactivity disorders (Scott 2000). The ICD-10 major diagnostic categories for disorders in childhood and adolescence are shown in table 8.2, chapter 8.

As in adults, the evaluation of the young person includes undertaking interviews where appropriate (see chapter 8) as well as the observation of behaviour. This includes response to separation from parent or carer, physical appearance including evidence of neglect or abuse, motor behaviour e.g. restlessness and hyperactivity, speech problems such as stuttering, or speech content abnormalities which may indicate psychosis or mania, difficulties in social interaction, and lastly, any evidence for affective disorder such as anxiety or depression. Behaviour and relationships at school form an important part of the assessment of psychopathology of the child or adolescent, and teachers are important informants. In younger children (i.e. those under the age of 9 [Angold 2000]), parents are also vital observers and informants. Where such different sources of information are available, it is expected that the agreement between them will at best be modest (Stanger and Lewis 1993, Reich *et al.* 1982), although this does not invalidate their veracity, since each informant provides a different view of the child's psychopathology.

Developmental psychopathology

The term developmental psychopathology, originally introduced in the 1980s, has been applied to the scientific study of how abnormalities can be understood in terms of the processes underpinning human development (Cicchetti 1984, Rutter 1988, Scott 2000). In order to evaluate delayed development, whether specific to certain areas of function such as reading or spelling, or more generalized as in those with Down's syndrome, detailed knowledge of normal development is required. Developmental psychology is the study of the normal ranges of development in healthy individuals. Since throughout childhood the individual is constantly changing, it is important that any assessment of delay is placed in the context of what is 'normal' and at what age (developmental milestones). For example, repetitive rituals may be normal behaviour in a 5-year-old but not in an 8-year-old. Similarly, language is acquired gradually, from the first words around age 1 year, to increasingly complex sentence and grammatical construction up to the age of 5 years (Yule 2000). Individuals who have language development that does not meet these 'milestones' are considered to have delayed language acquisition. In addition, those who have developed language may then stop speaking, and develop other behavioural problems associated with the autistic spectrum disorders.

Delayed development can also occur in relation to motor activity and coordination, continence both day and night of urine and faeces, and ability to interact and socialize at an age appropriate level, with peers and adults. The evaluation of developmental delay and other associated problems may require specialized psychometric testing which is beyond the scope of this book, but good accounts may be found in Shaffer *et al.* (1999) and Cicchetti and Cohen (1995).

Having considered the signs and symptoms of psychopathology in adults and children, we will now discuss the various ways these have been grouped together into syndromes or *mental disorders*. In chapter 3 we will discuss the different methods that have been used to classify mental disorders; taking a historical perspective to provide the background to current nosologies.

Defining and Classifying Disorder

Introduction

No classification which has been proposed can be regarded as all together satisfactory. This is partly owing to the fact that the true nature and limits of insanity itself have been imperfectly recognised. Almost every writer on insanity has suggested a special classification of its forms, and the majority have founded their suggestions either on the aetiology or symptomatology of the disease.

Blandford (1888)

Apart from the use of the old-fashioned term 'insanity', these comments, made over 100 years ago by an academic psychiatrist from St Georges's Hospital in London, sound shockingly up to date and familiar. In this chapter, we will describe and review the evolution of current international psychiatric classifications, namely the International Classification of Diseases, tenth edition (ICD10), produced by the World Health Organization (WHO 1992), and the Diagnostic and Statistical Manual, fourth edition (DSM IV) produced by the American Psychiatric Association

(APA 1994). We will examine how far we have progressed in overcoming the problems of defining and classifying disorder.

As we shall, see the main shift of emphasis has been towards naming and classifying diseases purely on the basis of symptoms and signs, and to steer away from categories of disorder based on their supposed causation or aetiology. This makes good sense in defining psychopathology, where, even though we may recognize general risk factors (for example a family history of the disorder, or exposure to unpleasant life events), for most cases of most disorders, the precise aetiology remains unclear. The authors of the *Diagnostic and Statistical Manual,* third edition (DSMIII)(APA 1980), were among the first to attempt an exclusively descriptive approach embracing all of psychopathology that was, as they put it, *atheoretical* with respect to causation. This can in part be seen as a reaction against the role of psychoanalytically influenced theory, in earlier versions of the *Diagnostic and Statistical Manual* (DSM) (APA 1968), and led to the abandonment of a descriptive term covering a whole broad category of disorder, the *neuroses.* This term referred to less severe disorders such as depression and anxiety, where insight was retained, and subjects recognize that there is a mental health problem, (as compared with the *psychoses* where insight was lost). The term *neurosis* was taken over by Freud, and applied in relation to psychoanalysis. The term then acquired psychodynamic connotations that led to confusion about what was actually meant, and hence it being dropped by DSMIII's authors. However such confusion did not occur outside of North America, and the term *neurosis* is retained in ICD10.

However, it is not possible to entirely ignore aetiology, since there are two main categories of disorders where the pathology is known. *Organic mental disorders,* such as acute confusional states and the dementias, can be shown to have a demonstrable neuropathology or associated metabolic disturbance. DSMIV, but not ICD10, attempts to avoid using the term 'organic' by introducing the category of *cognitive disorders.* Similarly, mental disorders that arise out of the misuse of, or dependence on, drugs or alcohol also have a known aetiology.

That said, the majority of disorders fall into the category of '*functional*', that is, in the traditional sense of being characterized by dysfunction with (as yet) no demonstrated cause or lesion. The functional/organic dichotomy is, of course, unsatisfactory. The history of psychiatry (and of medicine in general) has seen a progressive shift of disorders out of the functional into the organic category, as we will mention again in the next section of this chapter. However, for the present we have to accept that most forms of psychopathology remain 'functional'. Not knowing the cause of psychopathology means that it is not possible to confirm the presence or absence of disorder by the using any diagnostic tests. In other words, it is not possible to validate any of the current definitions of disorder. This issue of *validity* relates to most of the categories in current classifications, and to the methods used to define them.

As well as problems with validity, there are also associated issues regarding poor reliability, which in this context mainly relates to the agreement between clinicians regarding diagnosis. In this chapter we will first briefly examine the historical background to some of the main issues regarding classification, focusing on psychotic disorders as our main example. Second, we will discuss how to define disorders according to current concepts. We will describe the introduction of operational criteria as a solution to the reliability problem, and consider what operational definitions are and why they are used. Lastly, the strengths and weaknesses of this method of diagnosis and consideration of alternative approaches to measuring psychopathology will be addressed.

The historical background

It is worth noting that both psychiatry and clinical psychology are comparatively new disciplines. Psychiatry began to evolve as a distinct medical specialty about 200 years ago. (Interestingly, the term '*psychiatry*', although coined in the first half of the nineteenth century, and used in mainland European countries, was not used in English, even in medical circles, until about the 1930s). Psychology as a scientific discipline grounded in observation and experimentation, as opposed to psychology as a branch of philosophy, only came into being in the second half of the nineteenth century and clinical psychology as we would recognize it today is even more recent. The term clinical psychology was invented by Witmer, an American, in 1896. However, in Witmer's concept, clinical psychology had an educational emphasis rather than being a discipline with a major role in assessing and treating mental disorders. Modern clinical psychology as a profession only really arose in the mid-twentieth century, first in the United States, then in Britain and the rest of Europe (Miller 1996). Although growing in size and influence, in most countries it remains a smaller profession than psychiatry. Consequently the prevailing classification schemes that are in place today are based almost exclusively on a medical outlook, a model that contains categories of disorder rather than dimensions.

Indeed, even from ancient times attempts to classify mental and behavioural abnormalities have tended to be categorical. Classically these were considered to belong to four main types, the manic (excited, restless, irritable) the melancholic (gloomy, despondent, suicidal), the demented (foolish with failing memory) and the phrenitic (those suffering from delusions or hallucinations) (Hare 1990).

Although hospitals for the insane such as the Bethlem ('Bedlam') in London have existed since the thirteenth century, they were few and far between. The idea that people suffering from mental disorders should be treated (or contained) in hospitals did not become widespread until the late eighteenth century, and coincided with industrialization and large scale population expansion in the western world (Crammer 1996). Until then, those with severe mental disorders were generally kept hidden and often restrained at home. With increasing urbanization this was no longer possible and by 1808, in the UK, and Act of Parliament determined that 'asylums' should be built to house 'lunatics', as people with mental disorders were then known, in every county. Similar developments took place in other European countries and in the USA. Concentrating large numbers of the mentally ill in asylums, each of which was administered by a senior doctor, (called, in the UK, the 'physician superintendent'), meant that observations about the course and outcome of different patterns of symptoms could be made. Some asylums and clinics developed university affiliations, and this coincided with the expansion in the number of medical schools. This in turn facilitated a more systematic study of psychopathology, that led to a growth in knowledge about mental illness and, throughout the nineteenth and early twentieth centuries, attempts to refine and define categories of disorder.

However, nineteenth century asylums housed individuals with a somewhat different range of disorders than are usually seen by clinicians today. Many patients had disorders where we now know the cause. Such illnesses have become rare, because we have treatments or preventions based on knowledge about aetiology. These included general paralysis of the insane (GPI) (a late form of syphilis that can be prevented by treating the early or primary stage with penicillin) and, in American asylums, pellagra (caused by Vitamin B7 deficiency). However, other patients included those with what continue to be known as the 'functional psychoses', disorders that still have (mainly) unknown aetiologies. Throughout the early decades of the twentieth century, the asylums gradually emptied of those with treatable or preventable illness (such as GPI and pellagra), and those with functional psychoses made up a larger proportion of those remaining.

Academic or university based psychiatry became particularly strong in Germany as well as in France, where it was established around the turn of the nineteenth century by the legendary Philippe Pinel, and his followers such as Esquirol (Weiner 1994). The French have until fairly recently retained their own classification and nomenclature, but the rest of the world has, over the course of the past century or so, adopted a more Germanic outlook. The broad system of classification that has most influence even up to the present day is that proposed by Emil Kraepelin (1896) (Jablensky 1997) and was discussed in chapter 1. With regard to the functional psychoses, Kraepelin proposed two main categories (the 'Kraepelian dichotomy'). The first, *dementia praecox*, was characterized by an onset in early adult life (the 'praecox' part of the name) and led to deterioration of intellect and personality (or 'dementia'). Kraepelin separated these conditions from manic depressive insanity (now termed bipolar disorder) where full recovery occurred between episodes of illness (Kraepelin 1896). In defining dementia praecox, Kraepelin brought together three rather different presentations of the illness; *hebephrenia*, described first by Hecker in 1871; *catatonia*, described by Kahlbaum in 1868, and *dementia paranoides* which Kraepelin himself later added as a sub-type of his syndrome in 1913.

The name dementia paraecox was gradually dropped in favour of the term schizophrenia, as a result of Eugene Bleuler's influential work, originally published in 1911 (English translation published in 1950) *Dementia Praecox or the Group of Schizophrenias* (Bleuler 1950). This change of name, along with an apparently subtle shift in emphasis, turned out to have a marked and lasting effect on divergence of diagnostic practice, particularly between the USA and Northern Europe. We shall return to this problem again later, and to the influential studies that led to its resolution, when we come to consider reliability of diagnosis. However we will first turn to describe current classification schemes, and consider how they have arisen and what are their strengths and weaknesses.

ICD and DSM

The *International Classification of Diseases* (ICD), published by the World Health Organization, covers all disorders, not just psychiatric conditions.

A separate psychiatric section was first included in the sixth edition of the ICD in 1948, and the American Psychiatric Association produced its first *Diagnostic and Statistical Manual* or DSMI four years later (Cahn 1999). Until these publications, 'official' systems for the classification or nomenclature of psychiatric disorders had not existed. The two systems differed somewhat at their inceptions, with DSMI including considerable influences from the school of Adolf Meyer and tending to use the term 'reaction type' in preference to 'disorder' (see also chapter 1). Although the subsequent version, DSMII, included an attempt to align more closely with ICD8 terminology and its system of code numbers for disorders, there continued to be clear differences of interpretation. These were most marked, as we will later discuss, on the boundaries between schizophrenia, affective disorder and personality disorder (Cahn 1999). The really important paradigm shift took place with DSMIII, finally leading to a high degree of convergence of these two major classification schemes with the publication of the most recent versions (at the time of writing), namely ICD10 and DSMIV.

DSMIII, for the first time introduced an extensive and comprehensive set of explicit diagnostic criteria with every disorder given, in effect, an operational definition. (We will consider just what operational definitions are later). The DSMIII classification also incorporated another innovation, a multi-axial system of diagnosis. The potential benefits of a multi-axial system had been suggested previously and such a system was incorporated in an ICD9 schema for child psychiatry (Caron and Rutter 1991). However multi-axial schemes had not previously been widely implemented in any system of classification extending to adults. Altogether five axes were included in DSMIII, so that an individual could be assigned as follows.

Box 3.1 Five axes comprising the DSMIII multi-axial classification

Axis 1 – Psychiatric disorder
Axis 2 – Personality disorder (and/or mental retardation)
Axis 3 – Associated physical disorder
Axis 4 – Psychosocial problems relevant to the psychiatric illness
Axis 5 – Highest level of functioning in the year prior to assessment

---

The American Psychiatric Association (APA) revised the DSMIII criteria in 1987 (DSMIIIR) and again in 1994 (DSMIV). At the time of writing

DSMV is in preparation. The main DSMIV diagnostic categories are listed in Box 3.2. The code numbers assigned to the categories are broadly the same as those of past versions of ICD but (somewhat confusingly) ICD10 now has codes beginning with the letter F, followed by a number. This is because ICD10 covers all diseases, and F is the chapter assigned to psychiatric disorders. The main ICD10 diagnostic categories are shown in Box 3.3.

Box 3.2 Main DSMIV diagnostic categories

290.xx – dementias
291.xx – alcohol misuse disorders
292.xx – drug misuse disorders
295.xx – schizophrenic disorders
296.xx – mood disorders
300.xx – anxiety and somatoform disorders
301.xx – personality disorders (axis II)
302.xx – sexual and gender identity disorders
307.xx – eating and sleep disorders
309.xx – adjustment disorders

xx = fourth and fifth digit subdivisions

Box 3.3 ICD-10 main diagnostic categories

F00–F09 – Organic disorders
F10–F19 – Mental and behavioural disorders due to psychoactive
        substance use
F20–F29 – Schizophrenic disorders
F30–F39 – Mood disorders
F40–F49 – Neurotic, stress related and somatoform disorders
F50–F59 – Behavioural syndromes associated with physiological
        or physical factors
F60–F69 – Disorders of adult personality
F70–F79 – Mental retardation
F80–F89 – Disorders of psychological development
F90–F99 – Behavioural and emotional disorders with onset usually
        occurring in childhood or adolescence

A further contrast between ICD10 and DSMIV is that ICD10 and its components have been produced in several different formats that are tailored to specific circumstances. In particular, the authors of ICD10 were keen to differentiate between the needs of researchers, clinicians in specialist settings and physicians in primary care. Thus ICD10 includes a descriptive version, for use mainly by psychiatrists and clinical psychologists in everyday practice, the Clinical Descriptions and Diagnostic Guidelines (CDDG) and a version for use by researchers, the Diagnostic Criteria for Research (DCR10) where the disorders are defined operationally. There is also a shortened version for primary care (ICD10-PHC).

The ICD10-PHC was added because presentation of psychopathology in primary care and general hospital settings may be quite different to that seen in psychiatric practice (Ustun *et al.* 1995). The ICD10-PHC consists of twenty-four commonly seen conditions, presented in a 'user friendly' format, that includes the management of the disorder alongside the

---

Box 3.4 Conditions included in the UK version of ICD10-PHC

F00 – Dementia
F05 – Delirium
F10 – Alcohol use disorder
F11 – Drug use disorder
F20 – Chronic psychotic disorder
F23 – Acute psychotic illness
F31 – Bipolar disorder
F32 – Depression
F40 – Phobic disorder
F41 – Panic disorder
F41.1 – Generalized anxiety
F44 – Dissociative disorder
F45 – Unexplained somatic disorder
F48 – Chronic fatigue
F48.9 – Chronic anxious depression
F50 – Eating disorder
F51 – Sleep disorder
F52 – Sexual disorder (male)
F52 – Sexual disorder (female)
F70 – Mental retardation
Z63 – Bereavement

main clinical features (WHO 1996, Goldberg *et al.* 1995). The main conditions included in the UK version of ICD10-PHC are shown in Box 3.4.

The authors of ICD10 have also introduced several other innovations, including clinical guides or 'fascicles' covering those other elements of the classification of diseases that are not primarily to do with psychopathology but which are relevant to it. These include neurological disorders and disorders of the elderly. The 'family of documents' included in ICD10 is summarized in Box 3.5.

Box 3.5 The ICD-10 family of documents (modified from Cooper 1999)

Clinical Descriptions and Diagnostic Guidelines (CDDG)
Short glossary for the main ICD volume
Diagnostic Criteria for Research (DCR-10)
Short version for use in Primary Care (ICD10-PC)
Multi-axial schemas for (a) general adult psychiatry,
    (b) children and adolescents, (c) mental retardation
ICD10 Symptom Check-List
ICD10 Symptom Glossary for Mental Disorders
Clinical Guides (Fascicles) for (a) neurology, (b) headache,
    (c) cerebro-vascular diseases, (d) psycho-geriatrics
Lexicons of terms for (a) mental health, (b) cross-cultural mental health,
    (c) alcohol and drug disorders
An ICD10 Casebook
Explanatory documents (a) Understanding the ICD (b) Pocket guide to
    ICD10 Chapter V

One of the major differences between ICD10 and DSMIV is that the authors of ICD10 have considered that the needs of specialist clinical practitioners and researchers may be rather different and so have written two versions of the full classification: the Clinical Descriptions of Diagnostic Groups (CDDG) (also known as the 'blue' book) (see Box 3.6 for an example of the CDDG description of depression) and the Diagnostic Criteria for Research (DCR10) (also known as the 'green' book) (see Box 3.7 for the DCR10 operational definition of depression). The CDDG contains 'traditional' descriptive definitions of disorders, whereas the DCR10 contains explicit or operational definitions that are closely

Box 3.6 ICD10 Clinical guidelines for depression (WHO 1992)

F32 Depressive episode
. . . The individual usually suffers from depressed mood, loss of interest and enjoyment and reduced energy leading to increased fatiguability and diminished activity. Marked tiredness after only slight effort is common. Other common symptoms are:

a) reduced concentration and attention

b) reduced self esteem and self-confidence

c) ideas of guilt and unworthiness

d) bleak and pessimistic views of the future

e) ideas or acts of self-harm or suicide

f) disturbed sleep

g) diminished appetite

The lowered mood varies little from day to day, and is often unresponsive to circumstances, yet may show characteristic diurnal variation as the day goes on . . . For depressive episodes of all three grades of severity, a duration of at least two weeks is usually required for diagnosis, but shorter periods may be reasonable if symptoms are unusually severe and of rapid onset.

The categories of mild (F32.0) moderate (F32.1) and severe (F32.2) depressive episodes . . . should be used only for a single (first) episode. Further depressive episodes should be classified under one of the subdivisions of recurrent depressive disorder (F33).

These grades of severity are specified to cover a wide range of clinical states that are encountered in different types of psychiatric practice. Individuals with mild depressive episodes are common in primary care and general medical settings, whereas psychiatric inpatient units deal largely with patients suffering from the severe grades . . . Differentiation between mild, moderate and severe depressive episodes rests upon a complicated clinical judgement that involves the number, type and severity of symptoms present. The extent of ordinary social and work activities is often a useful guide to the likely degree of severity of the episode, but individual, social and cultural influences that disrupt the smooth relationship between the severity of symptoms and social performance are sufficiently common and powerful to make it unwise to include social performance amongst the essential criteria of severity . . .

Includes: single episodes of depressive reaction, major depression (without psychotic symptoms), psychogenic depression or reactive depression

---

Box 3.7 ICD10 operational definition for depressive episode (WHO 1993)

G1. The depressive episode should have lasted for at least 2 weeks.

G2. There have been no hypomanic or manic symptoms sufficient to meet the criteria for hypomanic or manic episode (F30) at any time during the individual's life.

G3. The episode is not attributable to psychoactive substance use (F10–F19) or to any organic mental disorder (F00–F09).

A. The general criteria (G1–G3) for depressive episode must be met.

B. At least two of the following three symptoms must be present:

    (1) depressed mood to a degree that is definitely abnormal for the individual, present most of the day and almost every day, largely uninfluenced by circumstances for at least 2 weeks;

    (2) loss of interest or pleasure in activities that are usually pleasurable;

    (3) decreased energy or increased fatiguability

C. Additional symptom or symptoms from the following list should also be present (for 'mild' to total 4 in all, for 'moderate' to total 6 and for 'severe' to total 8)

    (1) loss of confidence or self-esteem.

    (2) unreasonable feelings of self reproach or excessive and inappropriate guilt.

    (3) recurrent thoughts of death or suicide or any suicidal behaviour.

    (4) complaints or evidence of diminished ability to think or concentrate such as indecisiveness or vacillation;

    (5) change in psychomotor activity, with agitation or retardation (either subjective or objective);

    (6) sleep disturbance of any type;

    (7) change in appetite (decrease or increase) with corresponding weight change.

A fifth character may be used to specify the presence or absence of a 'somatic syndrome'.

similar in format to the definitions of disorder that are found throughout DSMIV (see Box 3.8 for the DSMIV operational definition of depression). How has this difference has arisen, and what are the strengths
and weaknesses of the two approaches? An attempt to find answers
to these questions is again helped by examining the recent historical
background.

Box 3.8 DSMIV operational criteria for major depressive disorder (296) (APA 1994)

A. Five (or more) of the following symptoms have been present during
the same 2-week period and represent a change from previous functioning; at least one of the symptoms is either i) depressed mood or
ii) loss of interest or pleasure.

(1) depressed mood most of the day, nearly every day . . .

(2) markedly diminished interest or pleasure in all or almost all
activities most of the day, nearly every day..

(3) significant weight loss or weight gain . . . or decrease or increase
in appetite nearly every day . . .

(4) insomnia or hypersomnia nearly every day

(5) psychomotor agitation or retardation nearly every day

(6) fatigue or loss of energy nearly every day

(7) feelings of worthlessness or excessive or inappropriate guilt
nearly every day

(8) diminished ability to think or concentrate or indecisiveness,
nearly every day

(9) recurrent thoughts of death, recurrent suicidal ideation without
specific plan or a suicide attempt or a specific plan for commit-
ting suicide.

B. The symptoms do not meet criteria for a mixed episode.

C. The symptoms cause clinically significant distress or impairment
in social, occupational or other important areas of functioning.

D. The symptoms are not due to direct physiological effects of a substance or a general medical condition.

E. The symptoms are not better accounted for by bereavement.

Problems of reliability and the need for new approaches to defining disorder

We noted earlier that for much of the middle years of the twentieth century American psychiatry tended to follow a more Bleulerian view of psychosis, and took a more psychoanalytically influenced approach to psychopathology generally than was the case in Europe. A further important ingredient in American psychiatry was the view put forward by Adolf Meyer that the differences in the subjective experiences and the presentation of symptoms between individuals were as large and important as the similarity within diagnostic groups. As we have mentioned earlier, this led to many of the categories in the first version of DSM being called 'reaction types' rather than disorders. However the trends in diagnostic practice in the USA were far from uniform, with some clinicians taking a more typically Kraepelinian approach. This divergence eventually led to substantial differences in first admission rates for categories such as schizophrenia in different states. The possible reasons for these diagnostic discrepancies were investigated in a study by Beck and colleagues in 1962 (Beck *et al.* 1962). In this study, 153 outpatients were evaluated by four Board Certified psychiatrists who undertook separate interviews of the patients on the same day. Agreement for the specific diagnosis was only obtained in 59% of the subjects. The major cause of the disagreement was considered to be the inadequacy of the nomenclature, which at that time was still the first DSM.

Subsequently, when transatlantic comparisons of first admission rates for schizophrenia and manic-depressive illness in were made, huge differences were found, with the schizophrenia appearing to be many times as common in New York as in London (Kramer 1961). This led to a series of studies entitled the 'US/UK Diagnostic Series' being undertaken (Kramer 1961). These studies evaluated diagnostic inconsistencies cross nationally. Project teams in Washington and London used a standardized interviewing approach and a computerized scoring system to produce a project diagnosis. These project diagnoses were then compared with the local hospital diagnosis in each case. The hospital diagnoses assigned by local psychiatrists showed the by now familiar national differences between the rates of schizophrenia and manic depressive disorder in each site, while the project diagnoses showed similar rates for these disorders in the two sites. The use of a structured interview and a standardized diagnostic procedure greatly improved diagnostic agreement.

Following on from there a wider investigation examined cross-national diagnostic practice in a range of countries. The International Pilot Study of Schizophrenia (IPSS) (WHO 1973) included 1,202 patients in 9 countries, the US, UK, USSR, Denmark, Formosa, Nigeria, Czechoslovakia, Columbia and India. As before, each patient received a clinical diagnosis from their local hospital psychiatrist and a project diagnosis via the structured interview, which was scored by a computer program. In seven of the nine countries the clinical diagnosis was consistent and mainly agreed with the project diagnosis. However, in the US and USSR sites the local clinical diagnosis was very different, although for different reasons. Whereas in the US the boundaries of schizophrenia had been greatly broadened by a combination of post Bleulerian, psychoanalytic and Meyerian influences, the Soviet era Russian psychiatrists were influenced by Snezhnevsky's concept of 'sluggish schizophrenia' (Tomov 1999). The diagnosis of the sluggish sub-type required no positive psychotic symptoms and included individuals with socially or politically unconventional ideas. (It was later shown to be the commonest 'diagnosis' in the notorious Soviet era abuse of psychiatric hospitals and was used to incarcerate political dissidents.)

As we have just noted, the US/UK series and IPSS achieved reliable project diagnoses using standardized interview backed up by computer 'diagnoses'. Essentially this requires that diagnoses are formulated as a series of explicit algorithms. Such an approach is rather different from standard clinical practice at that time which, as we have seen, relied exclusively on a description of disorders to which the clinician referred and made a judgement as to which patients fitted with what categories. The measures that were actually taken in US/UK series and the International Pilot Study paralleled and coincided with an approach to the problem of providing reliable diagnoses in psychiatry that was being proposed from a more theoretical perspective, namely the use of operational definitions.

Operational definitions

The use of an operational approach to defining scientific concepts originated from Bridgman, a physicist, in 1927. Bridgman stated that

> An operational definition of a scientific term S, is a stipulation to the effect that S is to apply to all and only those cases for which performance of the test operation T, yields the specific outcome O.

To paraphrase this, Bridgman is merely stating that to define S one needs to set up a series of experiments, the outcome of which is predicted. If predicted outcome occurs for the complete set of such experiments then the definition of S is fulfilled. In 1961 Hempel, a philosopher, suggested that the use of operational definitions could be applied to overcome the diagnostic difficulties in psychiatry. However, Hempel suggested that Bridgman's original definition should be modified specifically for psychiatry, so that:

> The diagnosis S should be applied to all of those and only those, manifesting the characteristic or satisfying the criterion O, subject to the proviso that O should be 'objective' and 'intersubjectively certifiable' and not something experienced intuitively or empathetically by the examiner.

The point that Hempel was making is that in psychiatric classification a range of clinical features, none of which are sufficient in their own right, should be required to make the diagnosis. Hempel suggested that these are reduced to a single criterion O, and that graded traits should be converted to a dichotomous variable by imposing arbitrary cut off points. Thus Hempel suggested that the test operation that should be applied in psychiatry should be *does the subject exhibit this much of X?*.

The first definition of a psychiatric disorder that lent itself to being caste in an operational format was that originally proposed by Schneider, for schizophrenia. Schneider proposed that any one of a list of what he termed *first rank symptoms* (FRS) was diagnostic of schizophrenia providing it occurred in the absence of 'coarse brain disease' (e.g. an obvious brain lesion or metabolic disturbance) (see Box 3.5). Schneider originally published his first rank symptoms in German in 1939 and translated into English in 1959. They hence predated by some way the debate on the introduction of explicit and reliable criteria. The FRS are well circumscribed and easy to define. Nearly all studies show that they allow very high inter-rater agreement, and they have had considerable impact on the diagnosis of schizophrenia throughout Europe and subsequently in United States. Indeed the symptoms are often incorporated in other authors' operational criteria.

The first operational criteria to be published *de novo* were the St Louis criteria (Feighner *et al.* 1972) (also known as the Feighner criteria). Interestingly, although these criteria provide definitions for schizophrenia and affective disorder that are recognizably and fairly precisely operational in structure as defined by Hempel, the St Louis group neither cited Hempel's

---

Box 3.9 Schneider's first rank symptom of Schizophrenia in the form of an operational definition

A. Absence of coarse brain disease

B. One or more of:

- Thoughts inserted
- Thoughts withdrawn
- Thoughts broadcast

- Thoughts spoken aloud (voice echoes thoughts)
- Third person voices (voices arguing about or discussing subject)
- Running commentary voices

- Made actions or impulses
- Made sensations
- Made emotions

- Primary delusional perception

A and B required for the diagnosis

---

writing nor used the term 'operational'. Indeed the practical attractions of the St Louis criteria proved to be more influential than any theorizing about diagnostic processes, and soon after their publication a number of other operational criteria were produced. The Carpenter criteria for schizophrenia (Carpenter *et al.* 1973) were selected following the analysis of data from the International Pilot Study of Schizophrenia. The Research Diagnostic Criteria for schizophrenia and affective disorder were first published by Spitzer and colleagues in 1975 and were subsequently revised in 1978. Similarly Taylor and Abrams's criteria for schizophrenia were also first published in 1975 and subsequently revised in 1978.

Operational criteria for psychiatric disorders were at first sometimes rather disparagingly termed the 'Chinese menu' approach to diagnosis. However, the St Louis and the Research Diagnostic Criteria in particular had a very considerable influence on the format of the criteria, later extending to the whole range of disorders in the *Diagnostic Statistical Manual* third edition (DSMIII) published in 1980 by the American Psychiatric Association. The publication of the DSMIII was a watershed in introducing a new, more explicit approach to diagnoses in psychiatry throughout North America and subsequently the rest of the world.

Strengths and weaknesses of the operational approach to psychiatric diagnosis

The strength of operational criteria is that they are highly reliable. Two or more raters who have received some training in the application of the criteria can obtain very good agreement about the presence or absence of the individual items as well as the overall diagnostic category.

Operational criteria are also so easily applied, and it is quite possible to construct structured interviews based on the criteria items. Over the past two decades they have received international acceptance, and there is now a well-established research base, which includes their application.

However there are a number of weaknesses and problems associated with their application. Firstly they are 'top down' in that the rules for their application are predetermined. Consequently the diagnosis cannot be applied to those individuals who nearly but do not quite fulfil all of the criteria. The various authors of operational criteria have usually got round this problem by including a 'rag bag' category such as 'atypical' disorder or a disorder 'not otherwise specified'.

Operational criteria are also somewhat two dimensional, in that the rules for their application usually only include fairly obvious features of psychopathology. In the case of schizophrenia this means items such as delusions and hallucinations. Important clinical detail such as family history, pre-morbid functioning, past response to and compliance with medication are not included in most operational definitions. Similarly, more nebulous or difficult to rate items such as the negative symptoms of schizophrenia are often not included.

The DSM criteria not only direct research activity within the US, but are also essential in clinical practice. Insurance cover for patients and payment to physicians requires the assignment of a DSM category, and if the DSM system is not used insurance companies do not pay doctors. Consequently all psychiatrists in the US are required to accept the operational criteria as written in the most recent version of the manual, whether they agree with this clinically or not. We have previously suggested (Farmer *et al.* 1991) that this could lead to what we have called '*Procrustian bed errors*'. Procrustes was an innkeeper of ancient Greek legend who required all his visitors to exactly fit in his special bed. To this end he either cut their legs off or stretched them to ensure the fit! We have stated that there could be a tendency to ensure the 'fit' of operational definitions by 'stretching' or 'cutting' the number or type of the subjects' symptoms, to ensure that the correct diagnosis is produced and therefore payment forthcoming.

Despite these misgivings, nevertheless, in just over two decades operational definitions of psychiatric disorder have taken over psychiatric classification and psychiatric practice within the United States.

Also in spite of these limitations, operational definitions are now universally accepted as the method for assigning a diagnosis in psychiatry. It is virtually mandatory for research on clinical subjects to use one of the sets of operational criteria to define diagnostic groups. As operational definitions of disorder have had a major impact on the reliability of diagnosis, we will now consider statistical methods for evaluating reliability and validity in the next chapter.

CHAPTER 4

Validity, Reliability, and Utility

Indirect and direct methods of assessment for evaluating psychopathology

As we have already discussed, in much of the assessment of psychopathology the focus is on internal, unobservable processes of which there is only indirect evidence. In chapter 2, we described the signs and symptoms that comprise the main types of psychopathology. We mentioned that in addition to complaints of subjective distress (symptoms), evidence for the presence of psychopathology may also be shown in the form of abnormal behaviour, which may be self-reported by the subject or observed by a clinician/researcher or other informant (observational measures or signs). One such example of this type of evidence can be noted in the examination of children with suspected attention deficit hyperactivity disorder (ADHD). Evidence regarding a subject's ADHD could consist of both the individual's own description of their perceptions, cognitions and emotions and of observations by a clinician or, for that matter, by a parent or a teacher. Probably, the simplest way of measuring psychopathology is by the means of questionnaires. The subject or an informant/observer (such as a spouse, a close friend, parent or teacher) answers a series of questions about the subject's behaviour and experiences, either in a written pencil and paper or computerized form. Some examples of the use of questionnaires are given in more detail elsewhere, particularly in chapters 7, 8 and 9.

Another systematic way in which psychopathology can be assessed is via standardized clinical interviews, that can be structured or semi structured (see chapter 5). Here a clinician or researcher elicits descriptions of an individual's experience and their cognitive and emotional state. In some standardized interviews (Wing *et al.* 1990), the clinician's observations of the subject's mental state and behaviour during the interview is also part of the objective assessment.

Standardized interviews and, in the main, questionnaire methods arise out of a general approach that we have already referred to in chapter 1 as *descriptive psychopathology*. Evidence for the presence of psychopathology can also be based on an individual's responses to highly controlled conditions aimed at sampling specific memory, attentional, perceptual or emotional processes (termed neurocognitive or neuropsychological approaches). An example of this broad area of study, that we have referred to earlier in chapter one as *experimental psychopathology*, is the recall and recognition of episodic information to test memory processing in individuals with Alzheimer's disease (see also chapter 8).

It is worth pointing out that although psychopathology presents particular challenges for those engaged in devising methods for its measurement, it is by no means unique in this respect. Other branches of science also encounter problems. Take, for example, the measurement of temperature in the physical sciences. One of the main methods for assessing temperature consists of measuring the length of a column of mercury, from which temperature is inferred. Consequently what is measured is what temperature does, rather than what it is. Similarly, much evidence supporting the presence of psychopathology is about what psychopathology results in or *does* rather than what it *is*.

There remain a number of features salient to a variety of measures that require more general discussion and these will be addressed here. In chapter 3, we described the major problems relating to the disagreements between psychiatrists over diagnosis. This diagnostic inconsistency was not trivial and led to major differences in first admission rates for schizophrenia and manic-depressive illness between the US and the UK. The introduction of operational definitions of mental disorder was one attempt to improve diagnostic precision. However, problems relating to validity and reliability, continue to preoccupy those researching mental disorders. Before considering more specifically the methods for measuring psychopathology, we will discuss the more general issues relating to validity, reliability and utility.

The preferred properties of measurement tools

How do we assess the properties of measures of psychopathology? To answer this, we need to start by asking a number of general questions that apply to every instrument of measurement. First, is the instrument measuring what it sets out to measure – is it a *valid* measure? Second, does it measure consistently – is it *reliable*? Finally, is the measure useful, does it work, is it suitable for the purpose of the enquiry? – Has it *utility*? As we have intimated in other chapters, there are problems in assessing some of these psychometric properties in measures of psychopathology, and in this respect, there is no doubt that the assessment of validity poses the greatest difficulties. This chapter will describe both how we assess validity, reliability and utility of measures of psychopathology as well as address their limitations.

Validity

The concept of validity can be approached from a number of aspects. Validity has been described as consisting of the following forms or types, *Face, Content, Criterion, Concurrent, Predictive and Construct*. The first two types, face and content validity, are necessary starting points for any measure but, it could be argued, depend considerably on subjective judgements. The other forms, criterion, concurrent, predictive and construct validity, incorporate objective components into their assessment.

Face validity describes whether the measure appears to test what it sets out to test. At best it is a 'common sense' assessment of validity. For example, a measure of psychotic symptoms should include questions on hallucinations, delusions and thought disorder and a measure of depressed mood should include questions on dysphoria, irritability, concentration, sleep and weight disturbance. It is often desirable not to stop there, and use face validity on its own, but to attempt a combination with other more objective means of assessing overall validity.

Content validity, as the name suggests, this refers to whether the specific content of the measure provides a comprehensive and balanced assessment. Thus, in addition to including items that at face level represent psychotic or depressive features, the measures should possess a sufficient range of questions relating to psychosis or depression. In addition, the weighting between items should be balanced in proportion to their relevance. As with face validity, it is desirable to combine content validity with more objective methods.

Criterion validity refers to the agreement between a measure and an alternative, independent measure of the same construct. If there is significant agreement, the second test is seen as measuring the same factor or factors as the first or independent procedure. If there is little agreement, the test may have value but is not equivalent to the original procedure. For example, Dyson and colleagues (1998) studied the criterion validity of several drug and alcohol scales, which included the four item CAGE questions (Ewing 1984) (see also chapter 7). Each of these tests was compared to a diagnosis of alcohol and drug abuse based on the structured clinical interview for DSM-III- R (SCID) (Spitzer *et al.* 1992), which acted as the criterion reference. Dyson and colleagues (1998) found that the short screening scales were valid in the sense that they accurately detected cases where a diagnosis of substance abuse had been assigned using the more thorough and time consuming SCID interview.

Criterion validity can further be divided into concurrent and predictive validity. An instrument is said to have concurrent validity when it shows agreement with the criterion measure, when both measures are given at the same time. Predictive validity reflects the ability of an instrument to predict the values of a future criterion reference measure. For example, assessing the predictive validity of a test of scholastic aptitude for prospective medical students, one would compare their test results with their success in medical school. In most cases, the most scientifically useful test is one that can predict future behaviour, and thus in general predictive accuracy is a more important aspect of validity than is concurrent agreement.

Statistical considerations

The statistical measures used to test criterion validity depend on the type of data. If both the assessment and criterion measure are continuously distributed, then one has the choice of either Pearson's product-moment correlation coefficient, if bivariate normality can be assumed, or Spearman's rank order correlation coefficient for non normal data. Correlational analysis provides measures both of the *significance* of the effect and the *strength* of the effect. Conventionally an effect is significant if it would be expected to occur by chance less than one time in twenty (usually expressed as 'p < 0.05'). However, what is usually meant by saying that a correlation coefficient is 'significant', is that it is significantly different from zero. Usually one is also aiming for a measure that has a strong effect, for example in predicting outcome, as reflected in a high positive correlation, i.e. greater than 0.7.

If both reference and criterion measures are dichotomous, for example the possible outcomes are 'case' or 'non-case', then significance can be tested using a chi square test (or Fisher exact test if expected frequencies are small). Validity can also be expressed in terms of *sensitivity, specificity* and *positive* and *negative predictive value* (see also chapter 7).

Consider the following hypothetical example. A consecutive series of attenders at an out patient clinic were asked to complete the General Health Questionnaire (GHQ) (Goldberg and Williams 1988), while waiting to be seen by the psychiatrist who, 'blind' to the questionnaire scores, then completed a structured psychiatric interview. A threshold score was used to define 'caseness' on the GHQ, and a computerized scoring program assigned diagnoses according to DSMIV criteria from the psychiatrist's interview ratings. The criterion measure is caseness defined according to the DSMIV criteria while the new measure is caseness defined by GHQ threshold score.

The *sensitivity* of the new measure (GHQ cut off score) is the proportion of true cases correctly identified; i.e. $a \div (a + c) = 0.8$. The *specificity* of the new measure is the proportion of non-cases correctly identified; i.e. $d \div (b + d) = 0.6$. The *positive predictive value* (PPV) of the new measure

Table 4.1. Agreement between a new measure and a criterion measure

DSMIV Criterion measure	GHQ score New measure	
	Case	Non-case
Case	80 (a)	40 (b)
Non-case	20 (c)	60 (d)

is the proportion of patients identified as cases that actually are cases according to the criterion referenced measure; i.e. a ÷ (a + b) = 0.67. Finally, the *negative predictive value* (NPV) of the new measure is the proportion of patients identified as non-cases that are non-cases according to the criterion reference measure; i.e. d ÷ (c + d) = 0.75.

ROC analysis

Receiver (or relative) operating characteristics (ROC) analysis (see figure 4.1) allows validation across a range of possible cut off scores, rather than just a single sensitivity and specificity evaluation. In the example given above, a number of different threshold scores on the GHQ could have been validated against the psychiatrist's interview. In ROC analysis, the sensitivity is plotted against the false negative rate for a range of scores. A curve can then be drawn by joining the points together, which, where there is good agreement, should be convex, and close to the left side and top boundaries of the plot square. A ROC curve approximating to the lead diagonal from lower left to upper right indicates poor agreement between the new measure and criterion measure. The area under the curve is used as the index of the discriminating ability or power of the new measure. This can be calculated using the maximum likelihood method via a computer program (Swets and Pickett 1982) or by calculating and manipulating the Wilcoxon statistic (Hanley and McNeil 1983, Farmer *et al.* 1996). This approach is

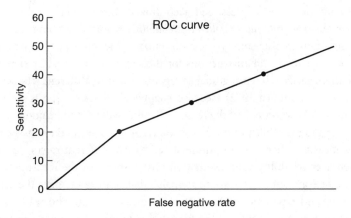

Figure 4.1.

particularly useful when validating screening questionnaires as it allows the optimal threshold score for 'caseness' to be determined (see chapter 7).

Construct validity

Construct validity is conceptually the most complex type of validity. It 'refers to the extent to which the construct that the measure seeks to address is a real and coherent entity, and then to the salience of the measure to that construct' (Prince 1998). In other words, in construct validity if a measure and construct are significantly correlated, this will support the veracity of the construct as well as the validity of the measure. For example, one may propose a hypothesis that the positive symptoms of schizophrenia are contributed to by abnormal inhibitory processes of attention. If a significant association was observed between a measure of inhibitory attentional processing and the positive symptoms of schizophrenia, then both the validity of the construct (positive symptom disorder as a specific subtype of schizophrenia) and the validity of the measure (the inhibitory attentional processing test) would be supported.

Reliability

Assessing the reliability of measures of psychopathology is, in general terms, more straightforward. Reliability reflects the consistency of the measure and is usually assessed according to three criteria: *inter-rater, test-retest* and *internal or split-half reliability*. Before describing these, it is important to note some basic requirements. Measures need to be constructed correctly, the instructions for their application must be explicit, and there needs to be clear guidance regarding severity differences between ratings (Wittenborn 1972) (see also chapter 7). If these aspects are not addressed, however expert the raters, reliability will tend to be poor.

Inter-rater reliability or inter-observer reliability assesses the consistency of a measure when used or administered by two different raters. Testing inter-rater reliability assumes that all other aspects of the measurement procedure are similar for each rater, also that both raters have the same training and experience in their use of the measure (Wittenborn 1972).

The problems encountered in performing tests of inter-rater reliability mainly relate to the comparability of test circumstances for each rater. For example, if two raters assess the same individual on a particular measure, the assumption is that they are testing the same thing. However, if the assessments take place too close to each other, the individual's memory of their responses to the initial rater may affect their responses to the second. Also if the two assessments take place immediately, one after the other, subject fatigue and the desire (conscious or otherwise) to hasten completion can lead to a lower positive response in the second test. On the other hand, if too much time is allowed to elapse between the first and second rating, then the subject's condition could change. Inter-rater reliability can also be tested, by having two raters rate the same assessment either by both being present at the same interview, or by the raters rating a tape or video recording. This process, if appropriate, can eliminate some of the problems that can confound the assessment of this form of reliability.

Test-retest reliability is also a coefficient of stability, which assumes that the trait being measured is fairly stable through time, or at least stable through the time separating measurements. Test-retest reliability thus tests the stability of a measure over time. The measure is administered to an individual or group on one occasion, and then following a period of time, is administered again to the same individuals. As with inter-rater reliability, it is assumed that other aspects of the administration procedure are similar at both occasions.

The statistical tests used to assess inter-rater or re-test reliability will depend on the situation and the type of data being measured. For continuous measures such as personality test scores, calculating an intra class correlation coefficient is generally more appropriate than a Pearson's product moment correlation. This is because intra class correlations are symmetrical in the sense that there is no independent (explanatory) and no dependent (response) variable. Rather what is being compared is simply the extent to which two independent variables agree. (This is in contrast with testing for predictive validity where what is examined is the extent to which a measure [independent variable] predicts a certain outcome [dependent variable]). For non-normal data, it is safest to rank both sets of variables and compute a Spearman rank order correlation. For categorical data an appropriate statistic is Cohen's kappa. The kappa statistic takes account of the agreement expected by chance and is not dependent on the prevalence of the condition in the population sample. However for measures with low population base rates e.g. number of cases of obsessive compulsive disorder in a general practise population, Yule's Y statistic should be used (Spitznagel and Helzer 1986).

Split-half reliability and internal consistency

For measures that are aimed to produce continuous scores relating to what is presumed to be a single dimension, internal consistency should be a goal. The assessment is made on a single administration of a measure, which can be split into two halves, which are scored separately and compared with each other. The test can be split into two halves randomly or by choosing alternative consecutive items. This form of reliability test overcomes many of the problems associated with test re-test and inter-rater reliability, but has certain limitations.

On the positive side, the conditions of test administration are very nearly identical for both halves of interest, as there is no time lag between administrations and the attitudes of the subjects should be nearly identical for both administrations. However, the test assumes that the items are sampling the same coherent construct and not a variety of independent factors. For example it would not be appropriate to carry out a split half reliability analysis on the total score a personality questionnaire designed to measure all of the 'Big Five' personality dimensions (see chapter 9). However it would be appropriate to divide up the items according to each of the subscales and perform a split half analysis of each subscale.

Arguably, a more comprehensive method for assessing the overall reliability and coherence of a continuous measure of psychopathology is by the examination of the measure's 'internal consistency'. The internal consistency of scales where subjects' scores consist of a summation of responses to 0,1 items can be measured using Cronbach's coefficient alpha. Cronbach's alpha has values varying between 0 and 1. An alpha coefficient between 0.6–0.8 is considered moderate but satisfactory and a score above 0.8 is seen as representing high internal consistency. Essentially, alpha is a measure of the degree to which each and every one of the items that make up a score agrees with the total score.

Utility

Choosing an appropriate instrument to measure psychopathology is dependent on the purpose for which it is required as well as its psychometric properties. Aspects of psychopathology can be sampled in a variety of ways, using any of a number of measures. For example, depressed mood can be measured by a self rating scale, such as the Beck Depression Inventory (BDI) (Beck *et al.* 1961), an observer administered scale such as the Hamilton (HAM-D) (Hamilton 1960) or as part of an extensive semi-structured interview such as the Schedules for the Clinical Assessment of Neuropsychiatry (SCAN) (Wing *et al.* 1990) (see chapters 5 and 7). If the purpose of the clinical or research enquiry is to quantify depressed mood as a continuous variable, with a view to obtaining a single measure of severity or as the starting point in assessing change over time, then the BDI or HAM-D is appropriate. Alternatively, if assigning a diagnosis (or classification) of depression is the primary focus, then a different type of instrument, for example a SCAN interview, would be appropriate. It is fair to say that within each category of measure of psychopathology (e.g. interview or rating scale) each available alternative has its own qualities and limitations that will dictate its relative utility. These issues will be discussed in detail in relation to specific measures in chapter 5 on structured diagnostic interviews and chapters 7 and 8 on rating scales.

Measurement scales

Measures of psychopathology can produce a variety of numerical outcomes. A *discrete* variable has a finite set of values, which are can be represented by whole numbers, (i.e. integers) not fractions. Sex (e.g. male $= 1$, female $= 2$) and social class (e.g. lower $= 1$, middle $= 2$, upper $= 3$) are good examples of discrete variables.

However, if a variable can take any value over a range of values, which includes a decimal point, it is said to be *continuous* (or a 'real' number). Examples include height, IQ and BDI score.

Superficially at least, 'traditional' of measures of psychopathology can be regarded as *nominal* or *categorical* in nature. Indeed much of clinical practice is concerned with assigning individuals to categories (see chapter 1). Thus diagnostic categories such as schizophrenia, bipolar affective disorder, unipolar depression disorder and generalized anxiety disorder, may be regarded as examples of nominal measurement. Strictly speaking the categories of a nominal scale should be mutually exclusive, but in practice in psychiatry there is often overlap or comorbidity between diagnostic groups, for example between depressive and anxiety disorders. Another feature of nominal scales is that there is no ordering of categories.

However one of the ways in which overlap between categories is overcome in classification schemes such as DSMIV is by imposing a *diagnostic hierarchy*. For example one of the exclusion criteria for recurrent major depressive disorder is that the episodes 'are not better accounted for by schizo-affective disorder, schizophrenia or other psychotic disorder' (American Psychiatric Association 1994). Thus in effect a diagnosis of schizophrenia 'trumps' one of major depression. Schizophrenia in turn, is lower down the DSMIV diagnostic hierarchy than psychosis (or delirium) 'due to the direct physiological effects, of substance abuse or a general medical condition and is excluded if either of these causal factors is present'.

The recognition of problems associated with diagnostic categories has, as outlined in chapter one, increasingly led to attempts to describe disorders as occupying a places on continua. Thus, depressed mood may be viewed as a dimension where severe depression signifies one extreme, but where there is nevertheless a continuum between disorder and 'normal' depressive symptoms or low mood.

Other types of measurement scales include *ordinal, interval* and *ratio* scales. Not only will these aspects of measurement affect the choice of statistical test, they also reflect the amount or type of information that a measure can provide.

An ordinal scale is a categorical where it is possible to introduce a rank order. For example the heights of twenty individuals can be expressed as their actual heights, or ranked according to the tallest (first) down to the shortest (twentieth). The ranking makes no assumptions about the magnitude of differences between categories. In the example given, the tallest individual may be two to three or only one centimetre taller than the second ranked and so on down the order. A special category of ordinal scale is the Likert scale (see also chapter 7). A Likert scale is when a graded approach is taken to the measurement of items, where the highest value is given to the most severe category e.g. a score of 3, the intermediate severity rating would then be scored 2, while the mild rating gets a score of 1 and if the item is absent then 0 is scored. The Likert scoring system simply summates the scores for all items. Another approach that uses the Likert summation of scores approach is when individuals are given a choice of replies to 'how much' the symptom has been present over the past few weeks, such as; 'very often', 'fairly often', 'once in a while' or 'never'? (Ilfeld 1976). With this method, 'very often' would be given a score of 3, 'fairly often' a score of 2, 'once in a while' scores 1 and never scores 0. Again scores are summated for all items. As with other types of ordinal scale, the Likert scores are simply a ranking, with no assumptions about the magnitude of the difference between, for example, 'severe' and 'moderate' or 'fairly often' and 'once in a while'.

An interval scale of measurement differs from an ordinal scale by have equal intervals between the units of measurement. Thus a score of 20 is seen as half-way between the scores of 10 and 30. The main advantage of this scale of measurement is that can be subjected to the basic arithmetic operations of addition, subtraction, multiplication and division as there are consistent intervals between each data point. The interval scale is therefore a truly quantitative scale of measurement.

An example is the *visual analogue scale*, whereby the subject is asked to place a mark on a line of standard length e.g. 10 centimetres, to indicate how much of the item is present. The ends of the line represent the extremes e.g. 'extremely depressed' and 'not depressed at all'. The number of centimetres from the 'not depressed at all' end of the line indicates how bad the depression is at the time of testing. Marks along the line at 2 centimetre distances can also indicate to the subject different degrees of severity of low mood, such as 'mildly', 'moderately', and 'severely' depressed. Using the visual analogue scale as an interval scale implies that moderately depressed is half way between mild and severe. In a study comparing the reliability of categorical and analogue scales, Remmington and colleagues (1979) showed that the levels of agreement were not significantly affected by the scale format, although they did note apparent differences in reliability depending on the statistic used. One potential problem about using visual analogue scales is that different individuals may adopt a different response set where some subjects typically use the whole range of the scale with others using only a restricted range of responses close to the middle. Where the aim is to assess change over several time points this can be corrected for by using standardized score. That is, the mean and standard deviation of scores for each individual is calculated and then each score is converted to a standard score by subtracting the mean and dividing by the standard deviation. This has the effect that all subjects have end up with mean score of zero and a variance of one.

The *ratio scale* has all the properties of an interval scale but with a true zero. The addition of a zero means that a score of 50, for example, can indicate twice as much of a given trait as a score of 25. Interval and ratio data can be analysed using parametric statistics.

Conclusion

We have described the methods for evaluating the validity, reliability and utility of measures of psychopathology. Further information about the statistical methods of analysis alluded to in this chapter can be obtained from a number of excellent texts (Dunn 1999, Armitage and Berry 1994, Everitt 1996). In chapter 5 we will discuss the development of diagnostic interviews for evaluating psychopathology, and describe the most internationally influential of these.

··

Diagnostic Interviews

Introduction

Although standardized interviews began to be developed almost half a century ago, the introduction of operational definitions of psychiatric disorders has seen a concomitant growth in the use of standardized interviews. To a considerable extent this is because using explicit definitions of diagnostic categories facilitates their incorporation into a structured or semi-structured interview format. In other words, it is relatively straightforward to take each individual criterion and formulate it as a standard question that can be asked by an interviewer.

In this chapter, we will consider interviews designed to cover a broad range of major psychiatric disorders and which are structured or semi-structured in their design. Interviews designed for more specific diagnoses e.g. personality disorders, substance misuse or subject groups such as children or the elderly, will be considered in chapters 8 and 9.

The interviews that we will cover in this chapter fall into two basic types. First, there are those that are highly structured and require the interviewer to ask every question exactly as it is written and in a prescribed order. The second type allows the interviewer to exercise a degree of judgement about how to order the interview and what questions to ask. While structured interviews can be readily taught to and administered by lay interviewers, the semi-structured interviews usually require the interviewer to have some clinical experience or prior knowledge of psychopathology. However both types can be shown to afford good to excellent reliability (see chapter 4). As in previous chapters we will commence by briefly considering historical developments. This will be followed by descriptions of the main traditions of diagnostic interview currently in international use.

The origins of structured diagnostic interviews

Although the introduction of operational criteria provided an important new impetus for their development, the first structured diagnostic interviews had already been used well before publication of the first sets of criteria (e.g. Feighner *et al.* 1972). As we have already outlined in chapter 3, two major international studies; the US/UK diagnostic series (Kramer 1961) and the International Pilot Study of Schizophrenia (WHO 1973) showed that the reliability of diagnosis could be substantially improved by standardized clinical enquiry and the use of computerized scoring programs. Indeed, one of the interviews used in both of these studies the Present State Examination (PSE) (Wing *et al.* 1974) was first developed in the 1950s. The PSE was widely used and a number of versions produced, culminating in the tenth edition, incorporated in the World Health Organization approved Schedules for Clinical Assessment in Neuropsychiatry (SCAN) (Wing *et al.* 1990).

Another major tradition in structured diagnostic interviews began in the mid 1960s with the publication of the Mental Status Examination (Spitzer 1966). A few years later, Spitzer and colleagues produced the Psychiatric Status Schedule (Spitzer *et al.* 1970), and two computerized scoring programs DIAGNO (Spitzer and Endicott 1968) and UPDATE (Spitzer and Gilford 1968). Both of these were designed to convert diagnoses to the (then) new nomenclature of the American Psychiatric Association, namely the *Diagnostic and Statistical Manual* second edition (American

Psychiatric Association 1968). In 1975, Spitzer and colleagues published one of the first sets of operational definitions for psychiatric disorders, the Research Diagnostic Criteria (RDC) (Spitzer *et al.* 1975a). These criteria are still widely applied in research, and along with the Feighner criteria, were highly influential in determining the definitions included in the DSMIII (American Psychiatric Association 1980) (see also chapter 3). To accompany the RDC, Spitzer and Endicott (1978) produced a new structured interview, the Schedules for Affective Disorders and Schizophrenia (SADS). The Structured Clinical Interview for Diagnoses (SCID), published in 1992, was produced to accompany the DSMIII-R criteria, and to improve on some of the limitations of SADS (Spitzer *et al.* 1992).

The Washington University department of psychiatry in St Louis, USA where the Feighner *et al.* (1972) criteria were developed, also had a well-established tradition, dating from the 1950s, of systematic interviewing, phenomenological description and the careful categorization of psychopathology (Robins and Helzer 1986). The Renard Diagnostic Interview (RDI) was developed around the time that the DSMIII criteria were published (Helzer *et al.* 1981) and covered the Feighner operational definitions of psychiatric disorders. The RDI became the forerunner of another important and influential series of diagnostic interviews, the Diagnostic Interview Schedule (DIS) (Robins *et al.* 1981) and the Composite International Diagnostic Interview (CIDI) (Robins *et al.* 1988).

Another early clinical interview, which pre-dated the introduction of operational definitions, was devised by Goldberg and colleagues to evaluate the milder types of psychopathology found in primary care and community populations. Devised around the same time as the self-report screener, the General Health Questionnaire (GHQ) (Goldberg and Blackwell 1970) (see also chapter 7), the Clinical Interview Schedule (CIS) facilitates clinical enquiry about the depression, anxiety and somatic symptoms commonly reported in community samples (Goldberg *et al.* 1970).

Some of these early interviews, like the CIS and PSE, have been modified and updated over the years and enjoy continued widespread international use (Araya *et al.* 2001). Other interviews were produced specifically to tie in with different operational definitions. These include the Psychiatric Diagnostic Interview (PDI) (Powell *et al.* 1985) (Feighner criteria and DSMIII), the Structure Psychiatric Examination (SPE) (Romanoski *et al.* 1988) (a semi-structured interview based on the PSE, but including items covering DSMIII), the Psychiatric Epidemiological Research Interview

(PERI) (Dohrenwend *et al.* 1978) (covering various psychiatric syndromes rather than specific operational criteria), and the Comprehensive Assessment of Symptoms and History (CASH) (Andreasen *et al.* 1987) (produced to assess psychopathology and produce diagnoses according to the DSMIIIR criteria).

Although all of these interviews have had their adherents and advocates we will discuss in more detail the interviews that in recent years and currently have had the greatest international use and influence in research; namely SADS and SCID, PSE and SCAN, DIS and CIDI, CIS and CIS-R. We will then conclude this chapter by describing two recent newcomers to the repertoire of structured interviews, the Diagnostic Interview for Genetic Studies (DIGS) and the Family Interview for Genetic Studies (FIGS) (Nurnberger *et al.* 1994).

Schedules for Affective Disorders and Schizophrenia (SADS) and Structured Clinical Interview for Diagnosis (SCID)

Spitzer and colleagues produced the first version of their own operationally defined criteria for mental disorders, the Research Diagnostic Criteria, in 1975. These were revised in 1978 (Spitzer *et al.* 1975b, Spitzer *et al.* 1978). In order to provide a standardized instrument to cover the diagnoses included in the (revised) Research Diagnostic Criteria (RDC), Spitzer and colleagues devised the Schedule for Affective Disorders and Schizophrenia (SADS) (Spitzer and Endicott 1978). A number of versions of SADS have been published, including a lifetime version SADS-L and SADS-LA, a version to provide more extensive cover of anxiety disorders and incorporate items to cover DSMIII criteria (Mannuzza *et al.* 1986). A version to measure changing psychopathology was also introduced (SADS-C).

The SADS interviews are very detailed and can take up to three hours to complete. Despite the use of a highly structured format, and the requirement to stick strictly to the order of the questions, the authors recommend that the interview is given by a clinician rather than by a lay interviewer. In practice what constitutes a trained clinician has been interpreted rather liberally by researchers, and studies have often used nurses or graduate psychologists as their interviewers. Training videos demonstrating how the interview is to be administered are available in various languages.

In order to provide a shorter, more interviewer and respondent-friendly interview, the Structured Clinical Interview for Diagnosis (SCID) was

Table 5.1. Diagnostic interviews in international use.

Name	Authors	What criteria are assessed	Type of interview	Approximate time to administer
Schedules for Affective Disorders and Schizophrenia (SADS)	Endicott and Spitzer 1978	All disorders in RDC. Revisions cover DSM and change in psychopathology	Clinical use and structured	Over 3 hours
Structured Clinical Interview for Diagnosis (SCID)	Spitzer et al. 1989	DSMIII criteria. Versions for no psychopathology and for personality disorders. Updated for later versions of DSM	Clinical use and structured	1–2 hours
Schedules for the Clinical Assessment of Neuropsychiatry (SCAN)	Wing et al. 1990	ICD10 and DSMIV criteria	Clinical use and semi-structured	1–2 hours
Composite International Diagnostic Interview (CIDI)	Robins et al. 1983	ICD10 and DSMIV	Lay use and highly structured	1–2 hours
Diagnostic Interview Schedule (DIS)	Robins et al. 1980	DSMIII in first version-updated for later versions of DSM	Lay use and highly structured	1–2 hours
Clinical Interview Schedule (CIS) & Clinical Interview Schedule Revised (CIS-R)	Goldberg et al. 1970 Lewis et al. 1992	Not tied to any operational criteria ICD10	Clinical use and structured Lay use and structured	1 hour 1 hour
Diagnostic interview for Genetic Studies (DIGS) and Family Inteview for Genetic Studies (FIGS)	Nurnberger et al. 1994	Feighner, RDC, DSMIII, DSMIV, DSMIIIR, ICD10 (also incorporates OPCRIT – see chapter 6)	Clinical and structured	2–3 hours

published to coincide with the publication of DSMIIIR (Spitzer *et al.* 1992). SCID also requires a greater degree of clinical expertise to administer and the inclusion of more 'skip out' instructions compared to SADS allows the interview to proceed faster. Like SADS, different versions of SCID are available. There are different versions for those who are assumed to have overt psychopathology (because for example because they are patients under treatment) and those who have no previously known mental health problem (for example those included in general population surveys). There is also a related interview known as SCIDII, which covers personality disorders in Axis II (see also chapter 9). Unlike other diagnostic interviews, SADS and SCID do not have computerized scoring programs, since the layout of the questions indicates to the rater when the criteria for a particular diagnosis are fulfilled.

More recently, Spitzer and colleagues have turned their attention to the evaluation of psychopathology in primary care settings. Their brief interview called PRIME-MD (Spitzer *et al.* 1994), for use by primary care physicians, is discussed in more detail in chapter 7.

Clinical Interview Schedule (CIS) and Clinical Interview Schedule Revised (CIS-R)

The CIS was devised to evaluate depression, anxiety and somatic symptoms commonly reported in primary care settings (Goldberg *et al.* 1970). Although the original interview was not 'tied' to any operational definitions of psychiatric disorder, a more recent revision CIS-R covers ICD10 criteria (Lewis *et al.* 1992). The original CIS was devised to be administered by a psychiatrist, and has been used extensively in epidemiological studies in different countries (Araya *et al.* 2001). In the 1980s, a self administered, computerized version was produced that showed good agreement with a standard CIS undertaken by a psychiatrist (Lewis *et al.* 1988). The CIS-R (Lewis *et al.* 1992) can be administered by trained lay interviewers. This interview, has been used in a recent large epidemiological study undertaken in the UK, the National Psychiatric Morbidity Survey of Great Britain (Jenkins *et al.* 1997). Shorter than some other interviews used in similar settings such as the CIDI, (and consequently less costly), it is still comprehensive in terms of its coverage of the main psychiatric disorders found in the general and primary care populations.

World Health Organization approved diagnostic interviews

Another milestone in the development of structured interviews was the World Health Organization's revision of the International Classification of Diseases (ICD) in 1992. As we have described in chapter 3, accompanying the tenth edition of the ICD clinical guidelines (ICD-10) for chapter 'F' on psychiatric disorders published in 1992, (WHO 1992) an operational criteria version for research was subsequently produced and published in 1993 (WHO 1993).

In line with these developments, the WHO and the Alcohol and Drug and Mental Health Authority (ADAMHA) in the United States, established a task force which had the aim of 'improving the accuracy and reliability of measurement and classification of psychiatric disorders' (Jablensky *et al.* 1993). The development of three structured diagnostic interviews which then became officially recognized for international use by the WHO was sponsored by the task force. These were the Schedules for the Clinical Assessment of Neuropsychiatry, (SCAN) (Wing *et al.* 1990), the Composite International Diagnostic Interview (CIDI) (Robins *et al.* 1988) and the International Personality Disorder Examination (IPDE) (Loranger *et al.* 1994). The last of these will be further discussed in chapter 9.

All three instruments have been translated and *back translated* into a number of different languages, subjected to field trials in a various countries and have been widely used in research around the world. The process of back translation is widely regarded as a useful safeguard where an interview is being used in a language other that the one in which it was originally written. The idea is that a native speaker of the second language who is not familiar with the interview retranslates it back into the original language, and the outcome is then compared with the original version of the interview. This is designed pick up any obvious inconsistencies in the translation, and hopefully any failure to render subtleties and nuances in the questions from the original to the second language. SCAN is a semi-structured interview designed for use with clinical populations, CIDI is a highly structured interview designed for use by non-clinical interviewers in epidemiological research. This difference in application ensures that SCAN and CIDI are complementary, not competing, interviews. CIDI is most effectively used in large epidemiological studies where interviewing costs need to be kept low. CIDI's great strength is that the interview can be reliably administered by non-clinical or lay interviewers, following a modest amount of training.

This gets around the problem that use of clinicians as interviewers makes such studies far too expensive. Also in parts of the developing world such professionally trained interviewers are simply not available.

SCAN, however, enquires more intensively into the severity and duration of each item and is clearly much more appropriately used in clinical populations where respondents are more severely ill. The subtlety of SCAN, particularly in its enquiry regarding psychotic symptoms, is one of the interview's major advantages. In addition, its 'glossary' definitions of symptoms and signs are detailed and almost amount to a short stand-alone text on psychopathology.

Schedules for Clinical Assessment in Neuropsychiatry (SCAN) and Present State Examination 10th edition (PSE-10)

The PSE had already evolved through nine previous versions before a radical further revision began to be developed in 1980, in part prompted by the need to incorporate DSMIII into its coding algorithms. Originally, early versions of the PSE were devised to examine the mental state for the month prior to interview, however, the tenth edition incorporated much more flexibility regarding the time frame of enquiry. Ratings could be made for the most relevant time for the research study or the subject such as over their lifetime, the most recent episode of illness or a representative episode. Another restriction of PSE-9 was that only a limited number of major psychiatric disorders were covered. With the tenth edition, questions relating to additional diagnoses such as somatoform, eating, post-traumatic stress and substance misuse disorders, were also added. This expanded version of the interview was renamed 'Schedules for Clinical Assessment in Neuropsychiatry' or SCAN.

In PSE-9, the CATEGO4 computerized scoring program incorporated a 'bottom up' method for assigning the 'most likely' ICD-8 diagnostic category. Initially the 140 items rated in PSE-9 were combined into 35 'PSE syndromes' and then further combined into 6 'PSE classes' (Wing *et al.* 1974). Finally a 'tentative' diagnosis was given. (The main author of the PSE, Professor John Wing, was quite clear that clinicians 'make' diagnoses, not computer programs, which merely provide guidance). The incorporation of coding algorithms for DSMIII criteria meant that the computerized scoring program for SCAN (CATEGO5) became both 'top down' and 'bottom up'.

Subsequent versions of SCAN have incorporated DSMIII-R (American Psychiatric Association 1987), and more recently DSMIV (American Psychiatric Association 1994). According to its authors, SCAN is 'a set of schedules for the assessment, measurement and classification of psychopathology and behaviour associated with adult psychiatric disorders' (Wing *et al.* 1990). SCAN includes an Item Group Checklist (IGC) which provides a means of rating information that is only obtained from case notes or informants other than the respondent, as well as a Clinical History Schedule. SCAN contains a glossary of definitions of each item, and as previously mentioned, CATEGO5, a set of computer programs for processing SCAN data, and providing output.

The purpose of the SCAN system 'is to provide comprehensive, accurate and technically specifiable means of describing and classifying psychiatric phenomena in order to make comparisons' (World Health Organisation 1992). In order to use SCAN effectively training is required, but in addition interviewers need to have some clinical experience. The main feature of SCAN is that although the interview is semi-structured, it retains the main aspects of a clinical examination. The aim of the interview is to discover which items of psychopathology have not only been present during a certain time frame, but also with what degree of severity. As the glossary states 'The examination is therefore based on a process of matching the respondents behaviour, and description of subjective experiences against the clinical definitions provided'. We have already described the details of this process in our introduction to chapter 1. The illustration regarding 'worrying' that we discussed was in fact, modelled on section 3 of the SCAN interview.

Section 6 of the SCAN interview covers depressed mood. The first question relates to the experience of being depressed and enquires, 'Have you been feeling low in spirits recently?'. While some people who've been depressed will relate to question, others will not recognize the experience and will talk instead about being 'blue', 'gloomy', or 'down in the dumps'. It is important that these synonyms are also presented to the respondent. If the symptom is acknowledged, the severity and duration of the experience needs to be evaluated. The rater has to decide whether the respondent's subjective experience of low mood compares to the glossary definition. If so, the interviewer also assigns a severity rating according to a three-point scale. For this, the glossary gives the following guidance. Criteria for rating (1) 'Brief episodes of clinically depressed mood may occur on their own or appear within episodes of elated mood. A criterion for rating 1 is a period lasting at least 2 days'. For rating (2) the instruction suggests that 'The intensity is variable; the depression is sometimes not very severe or even absent. The depression remains in the background but tends to come flooding back . . . ' With the most severe rating (3), the glossary states that the rating should be applied where; 'deep depression lasts for long periods of time without variation unless it is diurnal . . . It is very difficult for the subject to give their attention to anything else e.g. cannot be distracted by working harder, watching something interesting on television or other people's conversation'.

Although the questions given in the SCAN interview are helpful for eliciting each item, they are not obligatory. The rater may use any questions they wish to establish the presence and severity of each item. However, each suggested question has been well tried and tested over many decades and previous versions of the PSE, so it is generally much easier to just follow the interview as written. However the constant emphasis in SCAN training is that it is the SCAN *item* that is being rated, and *not* the reply given to the question. Other important aspects of the SCAN interview are first, that scoring '0' is a positive rating that the item is absent (i.e. if the question wasn't asked, or the respondent didn't understand, ratings of '9' or '8' respectively are made). Second, if there is uncertainty about the presence of an item or its severity, then a 'rate down' rule is applied. While this may lead to a loss of some sensitivity, application of this rule enhances inter-rater agreement.

The Composite International Diagnostic Interview (CIDI) and Diagnostic Interview Schedule (DIS)

In the late 1970s, the National Institutes of Mental Health in the United States identified the need for a large multi-centre epidemiological study of psychiatric disorders. This ambitious project entitled the 'Epidemiological Catchment Area Program' (ECA) was set up to identify incidence and prevalence rates of DSMIII defined mental disorders in the US populations and establish service use. Five study centres took part, and 15,000 subjects selected from household and institutional populations, were interviewed (Regier *et al.* 1984). Such a large study required a diagnostic instrument which could be used by non-clinical lay interviewers working mainly in respondents' homes. Although the ECA researchers considered using a number of interviews, (including SADS [Spitzer and Endicott 1978],

PSE [Wing *et al.* 1974] and PERI [Dohrenwend *et al.* 1978]), the decision was finally made to commission a new interview. Consequently the Diagnostic Interview Schedule (DIS) was produced for use in the ECA study. The team of researchers in St Louis USA who designed the DIS had considerable experience both in the development of research diagnostic criteria and diagnostic interviews (e.g. the Renard Diagnostic Interview, Helzer *et al.* 1981). Consequently, they were well placed to undertake the brief of producing an interview which could be reliably administered by lay interviewers and which was short enough to be completed in a single contact. Other requirements of the interview were that it should include both lifetime, as well as the most recent occurrence of each symptom. For episodic illnesses such as depression and mania, timing and symptom profile of the 'worst episode' was also required.

The DIS, as well as its successor, CIDI, requires little judgement from interviewers regarding rating, since questions are mainly closed-ended. Also, a series of additional questions are asked for every positive reply to the 'Have you ever had . . . ' question, which guides the interviewer regarding rating the item. These additional questions were incorporated into a 'Probe Flow Chart' (PFC) (see figure 5.1).

As the figure shows there are five possible positive ratings. If the symptom has been present but has been mild a rating of '2' is made. If the cause of the symptom is use of medication, drugs or alcohol the rating is '3', while '4' is given if the cause is a physical illness. A '5' rating is given if the symptom is caused by a psychiatric disorder.

In response to the WHO task force, the principal authors of the PSE and DIS, John Wing and Lee Robins, attempted to combine both the DIS and PSE in a 'composite' new interview, the Composite International Diagnostic Interview (CIDI) (Robins *et al.* 1988). Early versions also included questions to cover Feighner and RDC criteria as well as DSMIII. Unfortunately, this made the interview far too long. Although reliability and comparison studies (Farmer *et al.* 1991) showed that the PSE items in CIDI gave good agreement with CATEGO diagnoses produced by the PSE given as a 'stand alone' interview, the WHO task force made the decision to remove all these additional questions from the interview. Consequently, CIDI reverted to being a revision of the DIS, covering DSMIII diagnoses. Later versions covered DSMIIIR and DSMIV operational definitions.

While early 'pencil and paper' versions of the DIS and CIDI required interviewers to learn the sequence of questions in the PFC, the procedure readily lends itself to a computerized format. Consequently, the

Figure 5.1.

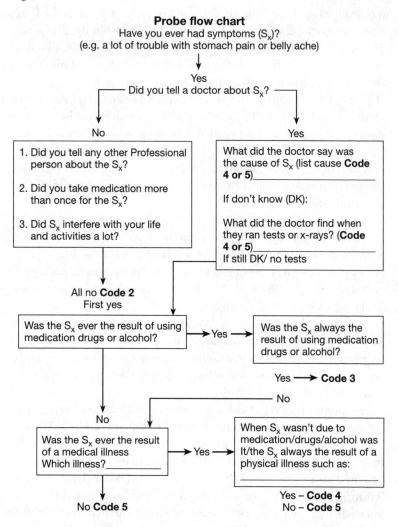

Probe flow chart
Have you ever had symptoms (S$_x$)?
(e.g. a lot of trouble with stomach pain or belly ache)

automated-CIDI, (CIDI-auto) (Peters and Andrews 1995) the comput-erized version of the interview, automatically displays the PFC questions in sequence. All that is required of the interviewer is to read them out to the subject and insert a 'yes/no' answer. As with SCAN, a computerized scoring program can also be used to score the CIDI interview.

Despite no longer being a 'composite' of the DIS and PSE, the CIDI has enjoyed much international application in epidemiological research

(Abou-Saleh *et al.* 2001, Spijker *et al.* 2001, Sandanger *et al.* 1999, WHO International Consortium in Psychiatric Epidemiology 2000). However attempts to find applications for the CIDI to assist the diagnostic process in clinical practice has been less successful. Two studies have examined the acceptability to patients of their completing the CIDI-auto on their own, in order to supplement the information collected at a clinical interview with a psychiatrist. Although the computerized interview proved popular with acutely ill psychiatric patients, their psychiatrists were less impressed; the conclusion being that the self-administered interview was of limited value in diagnosis and history taking (Rosenman *et al.* 1997, Komitz *et al.* 1997).

Subsequent developments: the Diagnostic Interview for Genetic Studies (DIGS) and the Family Interview for Genetic Studies (FIGS)

In part because of WHO approval, and because they have been translated into numerous languages, CIDI and SCAN and continue to enjoy international popularity in research .The SCID and to a lesser extent SADS continue also to have widespread use. Consequently most of the recent activity in devising new interviews has focused on instruments that serve specific types of research or special patient/respondent groups such as children or the elderly or those with eating disorders, substance misuse, or personality disorders where more specific detail about the illness is required than is feasible to include in general interviews. These are discussed in chapters 8 and 9.

We will conclude this chapter by briefly discussing two fairly recent additions to the repertoire of diagnostic interviews, devised for use in a particular category of research, genetic studies. These are the Diagnostic Interview for Genetic Studies (DIGS) and the Family Instrument for Genetic Studies (FIGS). Given the sheer volume of research being undertaken in the genetics of mental disorders, it is perhaps not surprising that some researchers in this field considered that a new interview was required, designed to meet the needs of genetic methodologies. Consequently, the DIGS was developed by the investigators from the sites participating in the National Institute of Mental Health (NIMH) Genetics Initiative (Nurnberger *et al.* 1994). The interview has drawn on the strengths of previous interviews and shares features in common with several of its major predecessors (Nurnberger *et al.* 1994). Designed to be administered by interviewers who are able to exercise clinical judgement when rating questions and who can also produce a detailed narrative summary of each case, DIGS is also poly-diagnostic covering RDC, DSMIII, DSMIIIR, DSMIV, Feighner and ICD-10 criteria for major psychiatric disorders. When using the interview, it is also possible to chart the course, chronology and comorbidity of illness.

Also included in the DIGS are the items from the OPCRIT polydiagnostic checklist (see chapter 6). These were added to ensure comparability between the NIMH Genetics Initiative and a similar multi-centre genetic study of bipolar disorder and schizophrenia that was being undertaken at the time in Europe (Williams *et al.* 1996b). The participants in the European study had agreed to interview using either SCAN or SADS, but all sites agreed to use the OPCRIT checklist in addition. This ensured that the final common pathway for diagnosis in the European and US was the same. (The next chapter will describe the OPCRIT diagnostic system in more detail).

The FIGS differs from all of the other interviews discussed in this chapter, in that it is designed to elicit in a standardized way information about the family of the subject rather than the subject themselves. The FIGS is given in three stages: 1) a pedigree is drawn and reviewed with the informant; 2) general screening questions are asked in reference to all known relatives; and 3) based on the informant's responses to the general screening questions, a Face Sheet and one or more of five symptom checklists (depression, mania, alcohol and other drug abuse, psychosis, paranoid/schizoid/schizotypal personality disorder) are completed for each first-degree relative, spouse, or other relative. A symptom checklist is completed if, based on the informant's responses to a set of general screening questions, the interviewer suspects that the psychopathology assessed by the particular symptom checklist is present.

The choice between structured or semi-structured interviews

There has recently been some disquiet that despite affording good within-study inter-rater reliability, standardized interviews have not always allowed good between study reproducibility. For example studies in the United States have yielded more than two fold differences (4% versus 10%) in the twelve month prevalence of major depression in the general population (Brugha *et al.* 1999a). These differences occurred in large scale epidemiological surveys and are unlikely to be attributable simply to sampling variation. Moreover the differences arose using highly structured interviews given in the main by lay interviewers and this has been interpreted by

Brugha *et al.* (1999a) as the root of the problem. Brugha and colleagues (1999b) compared the fully structured CIS-R with the semi-structured SCAN in a general population survey focusing on non psychotic disorders. They found poor concordance overall. This is in contrast with some earlier studies which compared the forerunner of the SCAN, PSE-9, with structured interviews such as the SADS-L (Farmer *et al.* 1993) or the CIDI (Farmer *et al.* 1987) and found acceptable agreement at a diagnostic, if not at an item by item level. These studies however included comparatively small numbers of subjects who were either hospital treated patients with psychotic or affective disorder or their relatives. It could therefore be argued that good agreement between the two types of interview here was dependent on there being a high base rate of clear cut, severe disorder among the subjects. This differs from the more usual, real-life situation explored by Brugha *et al.* which has the aim of detecting cases in the community and differentiating between shades of grey.

The advantages of a fully structured interviews are that in theory they should require less training, and because the scope for individual judgement is limited they can be administered by lay interviewers with no previous clinical or research experience in psychopathology. In practice, Brugha *et al.* point out that there is considerable variability in the amount and type of training that is given for most structured interviews, whereas there is greater uniformity for semi-structured interviews such as the SCAN, and provision of training is usually restricted to a limited number of centres. Although such restriction may be difficulty to enforce completely, the comparative complexity of interviews such as SCAN means that few researchers are tempted to pick them up and use them 'off the shelf' without training.

Brugha and colleagues regard the SCAN type of interview as administered by experienced clinicians trained in the interview as the 'gold standard' by which other interviews should be assessed. They found (Brugha *et al.* 1999b) that as measured against SCAN results the CIS-R gave low sensitivity (a low rate of true cases identified) but high specificity (a high rate of non-cases correctly identified) and therefore argued that actual rates of disorder are probably lower than the estimates that have arisen in some recent community surveys using fully structured interviews. They consequently propose that the way ahead is to consider abandoning fully structured approaches in favour of SCAN or similar types of interview acknowledging that, especially where non clinicians are the interviewers the effort and investment in training will need to be high. Taking a contrary view Wittchen *et al.* (1999) stress the value of standardized interviews. They reject the suggestion of

Brugha *et al.* that a major difficulty with fully structured interviews is the lack of scope for probing the subject's understanding of questions and the resultant need to take answers on face value. Wittchen *et al.* propose that such difficulties can be overcome by appropriate wording and construction of 'optimally valid questions'. This debate will continue but as will be evident to the reader from the first paragraph of chapter one of this book, we favour the probing approach so that the trained interviewer relies on a template that they have developed in their head rather than the exact words, and only those words, on a page or laptop computer screen.

CHAPTER 6

Polydiagnostic Approaches, Computerized Methods, and Best Estimate Diagnoses

The choice of diagnostic criteria
Precision with confusion
Polydiagnostic approaches
Consensus, best estimate, and computer generated diagnosis

The choice of diagnostic criteria

In chapter 3 we discussed the advent of operational diagnostic criteria which have now become universally mandatory in psychiatric research and, in some countries, most notably the United States of America, are also widely used in clinical practice. We have noted the limitations of operational criteria in chapter 3, but have also emphasized their great advantages and noted the reason why they have become so widely accepted: because they allow very good reliability in terms of agreement between two or more researchers or clinicians. This is a major advance over the previous state of affairs, where inter-rater agreement was pitiably low. Hence there is little debate over whether operational criteria should be used in research. The big issue is *which* operational criteria? At the time of writing, two systems vie for ascendancy – ICD10 and DSMIV. These, respectively, have the official backing of the World Health Organisation and the American Psychiatric Association. Although the two systems are not overtly in competition, most researchers feel that they can only choose one or the other. In practice,

Table 6.1. Percentage agreement and mean kappas for five sets of operational definitions (McGuffin *et al.* 1991).

	Agreement (%)	Mean kappa*
DSMIII	96	0.85
DSMIIIR	90	0.74
Feighner criteria	81	0.61
Research Diagnostic Criteria	87	0.71
French criteria	90	0.74

*$P < 0.001$ for all definitions.

because of the dominance of North American journals, the choice is very often DSMIV. There is also a *recency* effect with researchers believing that they should use the latest (most 'up-to-date') system, so that few people now use DSMIII and DSMIIIR is also been used decreasingly. However, there is no hard evidence that DSMIV is 'better' than its predecessors, and it is a matter of personal preference or perceived likelihood of having papers accepted for publication that tends to decide the choice between ICD10 and DSMIV, rather than any persuasive scientific data.

If we allow ourselves a longer historical view, as we have done in discussing the introduction of operational criteria, the problem of choosing between systems becomes even worse. Thus, for some disorders, particularly the major psychoses, the choice is not just between two, but between several possible definitions. Table 6.1 lists five different sets of operational criteria, together with typical measures of inter-rater agreement expressed as mean Kappa coefficients across all diagnostic categories. All five sets of criteria are acceptable, and, at a casual look, one might ask whether there is any problem at all, since whatever criteria are chosen there should be good reliability.

However, the real difficulty arises not in disagreement between pairs of researchers or clinicians, but in poor concordance between *pairs of diagnostic criteria*. This was first demonstrated in a classic study by Brockington and colleagues (1978).

Precision with confusion

Brockington and colleagues (1978) applied ten different definitions of schizophrenia to two samples of psychotic patients. These were a consecutive sample of patients who were admitted to the Bethlem and Maudsley Hospitals in South London (the final number in the sample was 119) and a series of 134 patients studied at Netherne Hospital near London who were previously examined in the US/UK diagnostic project. The highest agreement between sets of criteria was for Schneider's definition, based upon first rank symptoms (Schneider 1959) (see chapter 3) and a definition produced by the CATEGO computer program (Wing *et al.* 1974), used to score an early version of the Present State Examination (see chapter 5). These showed 72% concordance, reflecting the fact that the CATEGO definition requires the presence of at least one first rank symptom as sufficient (although not necessary) to achieve a diagnosis of schizophrenia (also discussed in chapter 3). However, the average level of concordance between one definition and all nine other definitions ranged from 41% for the criteria of Langfeldt (1939) to 14% for the definition devised by Taylor and Abrams (1978). Brockington and colleagues (1978) commented that the previous state of 'inarticulate confusion' in the diagnosis of schizophrenia appeared to have been replaced by a 'babble of precise but differing formulations of the same concepts'. These authors also found that some definitions such as the Feighner *et al.* (1972) criteria were 'too strict', in the sense that they classified a comparatively small proportion of patients who had a clinical diagnosis of schizophrenia as having the same disorder according to the criteria.

Subsequent studies suggest that the situation is even more complex, and that whether a set of criteria are 'broad' are 'narrow' is to some extent dependent upon the data to which they have been applied. Farmer *et al.* (1992) compared the results from two of their studies in an attempt to examine the relationship between different operational diagnostic criteria for schizophrenia. The data that they inspected consisted of the frequency of operational definitions fulfilled by 60 index cases from a twin series and 144 consecutive admissions to King's College Hospital in London with a broad diagnosis of psychotic illness. The results are summarized in figure 6.1. As we can sees the relationship between the different criteria of schizophrenia is complicated, and appears to be variable for different data sets. For the King's College series the majority of subjects were considered to be schizophrenic on the basis of having one or more first rank symptoms using the Schneider criteria, whereas in the Maudsley twin series far fewer subjects fulfilled this definition. With the exception of the Research Diagnostic Criteria (RDC) (Spitzer *et al.* 1978) which provided the broadest definition of schizophrenia in both samples, there was almost a reversal of the order of the frequencies

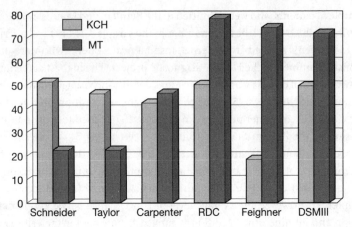

Figure 6.1. Frequencies (%) of subjects fulfilling criteria for schizophrenia in the Kings College Hospital (KCH) and Maudsley twin series (MT).

of the different criteria fulfilled in each data set. Thus, the King's College series was mainly positive for the Schneider (1959) definition, the criteria of Taylor and Abrams (1978) and the criteria of Carpenter *et al.* (1973). However, in the Maudsley twin series, the RDC, DSMIII criteria and the Feighner criteria were the most commonly fulfilled.

These differences cannot be explained purely on the basis of rater differences, as two out of three raters were the same in both studies. On the other hand, one of the differences was that the King's College series was selected on the basis of a broadly defined psychotic illness, where as the Maudsley twin series was selected by specifically concentrating on schizophrenia. On the other hand, this would not account for the low frequency of schizophrenia according to the Schneider criteria in the Maudsley twin series. Farmer and colleagues therefore suggested that the differences derived from two sources: first, the way in which the diagnostic information was collected and recorded, and second, from intrinsic differences in the clinical composition of the two series. In the Maudsley twin series the information was collected in a standard way according to a research protocol (Gottesman and Shields 1972), but without using a structured interview, and the principal researchers did not have a particularly 'Schneider orientated' view of psychopathology. By contrast, the King's College series was studied by a Schneider orientated group of researchers using the Present State Examination which, as we noted earlier, tends to place important weight upon positive Schneideran symptomatology.

The differences in selection of each series was that the twins were ascertained via a hospital twin register which accumulated cases over a period of almost twenty years. The King's College sample, by contrast, consisted of consecutive acute admissions including a portion of first episode cases. Therefore, it might be expected that the twin series would have a higher proportion of positives on those definitions of schizophrenia such as DSMIII and the Feighner criteria that require a longer period of illness, or where it is specified that a diagnosis of schizophrenia can only apply if there is failure to return to a premorbid level of functioning. Such criteria will therefore be fulfilled by only a minority of subjects in the King's College series.

The authors concluded that in the light of these findings, one needs to question the view commonly held then (and still held by some) that certain definitions of schizophrenia are particularly 'narrow' and 'strict' while others are 'broad' and 'liberal'. In the two samples that were compared, quite different patterns occurred for all sets of criteria other than the RDC so that for the Maudsley's twin series a definition of schizophrenia based upon Schneider first rank symptoms was narrow, while the DSMIII definition was broad. Just the opposite occurred in the King's College series where the Schneider's definition was fairly broad and the DSMIII definition was narrow by comparison. Thus, the results appeared to be crucially dependent upon the way in which the clinical information was collected and recorded, and in the way that the sample was collected.

Polydiagnostic approaches

A further problem, as discussed in chapter 4, is that reliability does not ensure validity. Researchers are faced with a bewildering array of different definitions of the same disorder and while, as we have noted, it is tempting to settle for most recently developed criteria or an 'official' definition such ICD10 or DSMIV, this risks the possibility of selecting a set of criteria that do not have optimal 'biological validity'. Thus, rather than choosing a single diagnostic system an alternative solution is to adopt a *polydiagnostic* approach where multiple sets of criteria are applied to the same subjects (Kendell 1982). The differing definitions are set up as it were in competition with each other, allowing a choice of the one that provides the most satisfactory validity.

Although this might seem to be a common sense pragmatic approach, it poses at least two major problems. The first is the familiar statistical difficulty concerning multiple testing. Thus, if some biological variable is measured and compared with individuals without a disorder and the disorder defined in multiple ways, the statistical significance levels need to be corrected for multiple testing. The second problem concerns the procedural difficulties of actually applying multiple definitions of the disorder in the same group of individuals. To try and overcome this potentially cumbersome exercise, the computerized OPCRIT checklist system was devised for research in psychosis and affective disorder (McGuffin *et al.* 1991). The core of this is a checklist containing the items from multiple sets of criteria for psychotic illness. In effect, 'top down' sets of operational criteria have been decomposed to their constituent items. The investigator is then able to proceed in a 'bottom up' fashion, where it is a relatively simple task to rate each of the item in the checklist. The computer program then reassembles these, using algorithms based on the diagnostic criteria. The operational definitions included in the OPCRIT system are shown in table 6.2.

A reliability study of the OPCRIT checklist gave satisfactory item-by-item agreement between three independent raters and highly significant levels of

Table 6.2. Operational definitions included in the OPCRIT checklist.*

Name	Author(s)	Disorders included
First Rank Symptoms (FRS)	Schneider 1959	Schizophrenia
St Louis Criteria	Feighner *et al.* 1972	Schizophrenia, mania, depression
Flexible system	Carpenter *et al.* 1973	Schizophrenia
Tsuang and Winokur subtypes	Tsuang and Winokur 1974	Schizophrenia subtypes
Research Diagnostic Criteria (RDC)	Spitzer *et al.* 1975	Schizophrenia, mania depression
Crow subtypes	Crow 1980	Schizophrenia subtypes
Diagnostic and Statistical Manual 3rd edition	American Psychiatric Association 1980	Schizophrenia, mania, depression
Farmer subtypes	Farmer et al. 1983	Schizophrenia subtypes
Diagnostic and Statistical Manual 3rd edition revised	American Psychiatric Association 1987	Schizophrenia, mania, depression
International Classification of Diseases 10th edition	World Health Organisation 1993	Schizophrenia, mania, depression
Diagnostic and Statistical Manual 4th edition	American Psychiatric Association 1994	Schizophrenia, mania, depression

* OPCRIT can be downloaded from www.iop.kcl.ac.uk/*IoP/Departments/ SGDPsyc/opcrit.stm*

agreement for diagnostic categories (McGuffin *et al.* 1991). The system was subsequently used in various epidemiological and genetic studies, including a multi-centre collaboration between US and European researchers, where it was shown that the approach gave good agreement at a diagnostic level across multiple sites (Williams *et al.* 1996b).

Another example of a similar approach, focused on a different area – attention deficit hyperactivity disorder (ADHD) in childhood – is the Hypescheme system (Curran *et al.* 2000). Here the problem that the authors have attempted to address is not so much to do with a multiplicity of criteria (Hypescheme covers just two sets, DSM IV and ICD 10) but with multiple co-occurring or *comorbid* disorders. Thus ADHD is often found in association with oppositional defiant disorder or conduct disorder, and may be comorbid with other developmental or neurological conditions. This has led to a certain amount of difficulty in comparing the results of studies in different centres. Hypescheme has been devised particularly to facilitate comparisons between molecular genetic studies and, like OPCRIT in psychosis and affective disorders, to serve as a minimum dataset in multicentre collaborative studies. (Hypescheme can be downloaded from www.iop.kcl.ac.uk/*IoP/Departments/SGDPsyc/hypeschemet.stm*)

As has been discussed in chapter 5, the majority of structured interviews used in psychiatric research have been developed with a top down structure whereby the interview is specially designed to arrive at a diagnostic classification according to specific set of criteria such as RDC or DSMIII. More recently developed interviews have tended to incorporate a greater degree of flexibility. Thus, interviews such as the CIDI and SCAN (see chapter 5) generate classifications according to both ICD10 and DSMIV. One of the most recently developed interviews for research on adults, the Diagnostic Interview for Genetic Studies (DIGS) is explicitly diagnostic, incorporating all of the items that are contained in OPCRIT, and therefore allowing patients with psychotic illness to be classified according to multiple different criteria (see table 6.2 and chapter 5). Essentially, authors of both OPCRIT and DIGS suggest that researchers do not try to use all these different sets of criteria at the same time, but rather that they choose one set as their 'lead criteria'. Subsequently, the other sets of definitions of a disorder can be used to compare with the results from other studies, as well as being used to compare definitions against validating criteria such as heritability and prediction of outcome or treatment response. Since the data are stored as items consisting of systems and signs, this type of polydiagnostic approach also allows the researchers to examine novel clusters of symptoms or dimensions based upon symptoms scores (Cardno *et al.* 1999).

Consensus, best estimate, and computer generated diagnosis

Commonly in research studies of patient or non-patient populations information is accumulated from a variety of sources. In addition to interviews these may include information from relatives or other informants, plus written material such as medical case notes. The question then arise as to how best to put all of the information together and arrive at a classification or diagnosis. The standard procedure has become known as the *best estimate* approach (Leckman *et al.* 1982). That is, the researchers involved in the study collectively review all of the available material for each subject and then arrive a *consensus* decision about the diagnosis. This pragmatic approach has a common sense appeal and would appear to be more reliable and, on the face of it, more valid than just relying on, say, interview data obtained and interpreted by a single researcher. Hence best estimate procedures are regarded by many as the 'gold' standard approach to arriving at a final diagnosis in research, but they are inevitably time consuming and costly. An alternative method is to devise a method of summarizing all of the available information in a way that can be fed into a computer and, since operational criteria should be readily translatable into algorithms, allow a computer program to 'make a diagnosis'. This of course is hardly radical since, as we have discussed in chapter 5, computer scoring programs have been devised for use with structured or semi-structured interviews since their first conception. The only difference in using a computer program as an alternative to the best estimate of a group of humans is that the computer input file becomes the final common pathway through which multiple sources of information are channelled. This is the approach which can be taken with packages such as OPCRIT or Hypescheme but it is also possible to do the same thing with, for example, the scoring program that comes with the computerized version of the Schedules for Assessment in Neuropsychiatry (SCAN).

Some recent studies have compared computer generated diagnosis with best estimate consensus. It has been shown that good to excellent agreement can be achieved between OPCRIT diagnoses and those made by best estimate procedures based upon the consensus of several clinical researchers (Craddock *et al.* 1996). It was therefore suggested that the computerized approach using the OPCRIT system may be used either on its own or as an adjunct to the conventional best estimate approach (Craddock *et al.* 1996). Taking a slightly different tack, Azevedo *et al.* (1999) compared OPCRIT diagnoses generated by an interviewer with those derived from an approach that combined both best estimate and computer diagnosis. In other words the consensus group made the decisions on the item by item input into the computer program. The results showed excellent agreement, leading the authors to conclude that the OPCRIT approach provides an efficient alternative to best estimate procedures.

This was of course a felicitous conclusion in the view of the present authors, but we appreciate the unease that many researchers will feel with a 'black box' or 'leave it to the machine' approach. Nevertheless, one logical consequence of using fully operationalized criteria for research is that the diagnostic method becomes purely algorithmic. Judgement is exercised at the level of deciding what signs and symptoms are present or absent but how this information is used is then automatic and mechanical. There is therefore a strong argument that at this stage computers that can be relied upon to give one hundred per cent reproducibility are far superior to even the best trained humans.

CHAPTER 7

Rating Scales: Screening, Observer, and Self-rating Questionnaires

Introduction

Rating scales have been widely applied in a variety of types of research. These include epidemiological studies, studies undertaken in particular settings such as primary care, or in subjects with medical disorders and drug trials where repeated measures of symptom presence and severity is used to evaluate response to treatment.

One of the first rating scales, devised to predict the later development of psychopathology, was used in the First World War to determine 'susceptibility to shock' (Woodworth 1919). Based on the idea of adding together the scores on individual items, this test was able to predict which front line soldiers would go on to develop 'shell shock' (also called 'war neurosis', and more recently called post-traumatic stress disorder) from those who would not (Winter and Barenbaum 1999).

However the serious development of rating scales to measure psychopathology did not occur until the last half of the twentieth century. Usually devised to address one particular research problem, the application of the more popular instruments has been extended into other research areas. This has led to modifications, shortening or different versions of the questionnaire being produced. For example, the Hamilton Depression Rating Scale (HAM-D) (Hamilton 1960) was originally devised to be an observer rating scale. Subsequently, Carroll and colleagues (Carroll *et al.* 1981) produced a self-report questionnaire modelled on the items included in the HAM-D.

Typically rating scales consist of a list of items relating to the type of psychopathology being assessed. These are completed by the subject (self-rated) or by an observer (clinician, trained professional or family informant). Originally devised as 'pencil and paper tests', it is now common to administer rating scales by computer. This is a convenient and increasingly popular approach which improves coding accuracy, because answers recorded on paper generally require subsequent entry on to a computer database, which can lead to transcription errors.

Rating scales fall into two broad types; those devised for screening or case finding and those designed to measure change in severity of psychopathology over time, although there are some scales which are applicable to both types of research. For example, the Beck Depression Inventory (Beck *et al.* 1961) can be used as both a screener (Beck *et al.* 1997) and to rate symptom severity over time (Beck *et al.* 1962).

Case finding in the general population

Finding 'cases' of psychiatric disorder in the general population, in order to estimate the prevalence and incidence of psychiatric disorders, requires the assessment of large numbers of subjects for the presence of psychopathology. In such settings, most respondents will not fulfil operational criteria for any mental disorder, but about a third will have minor or transient degrees of psychological distress (Goldberg and Huxley 1992) at the time of assessment. Most of this mild psychopathology consists of symptoms of depression and anxiety and is often self-limiting, but nonetheless may still cause distress, impairment and time off work.

While some large epidemiological studies have undertaken detailed diagnostic interviews with every respondent (Regier *et al.* 1984), in other situations this may be too costly or inappropriate. An alternative method uses a short but sensitive screening procedure, usually in the form of a self-report questionnaire, to determine which subjects are most likely to fulfil criteria for a mental disorder. This enables a subset of high scoring subjects to be identified, who can then be asked to participate in a confirmatory, diagnostic interview. The same screening questionnaires can also provide a range of scores whereby those who have less severe problems with their mental well-being can also be identified.

Two-stage sampling methods

In such two-stage sampling procedures, the population under investigation receives a short self-report screening questionnaire that can be sent by mail. In the second stage, more detailed interviews are undertaken on representative subsets of individuals. Typically, these subsets are randomly selected from across the range of scores; the results from the smaller number of interviews can then be weighted back to the total population (Goldberg 1981). One advantage of this method is that there is substantial saving of interviewer's time with little or no loss of precision (Prince 1998). One disadvantage, however, is that it can be difficult to track down or persuade individuals to participate in the second stage interviews, thereby reducing the representativeness of the sample.

Main requirements of screening questionnaires

The main requirements of screening questionnaires are that they should be easily administered, acceptable to subjects, short and objective, and that they can effectively differentiate between those who are psychologically healthy from those who are ill. While it is not necessary for screening questionnaires to differentiate between types of psychiatric disorder, it is important that more severe forms of mental impairment can be differentiated from less severe forms.

In community and general practice settings, psychological distress is not only caused by mental disorder but can also be caused by relationship difficulties or associated with aspects of personality. In order to narrow the focus and limit the number of questions, most general psychopathology screening questionnaires are targeted at psychopathology that caused a change in function or disruption to daily life, rather than the broad range of ongoing problems which may have been present for some time. Other self-report or informant methods (see chapter 9) methods can be used to evaluate personality or the quality of interpersonal relationships.

As we have previously discussed in chapter 1 and elsewhere, psychological disturbance can be thought of as being distributed throughout the population along a continuum of severity. Consequently, there is not a sharp distinction between 'cases' of mental disorder and supposedly 'normal' individuals (Goldberg and Williams 1988), and scores on a screening questionnaire can therefore be considered as giving a probability estimate of an individual having a psychiatric disorder. In other words, compared to an independent psychiatric assessment, the 'threshold score' on a screening questionnaire is the score at which the probability that any individual will have a disorder exceeds one half (Goldberg and Williams 1988).

It is possible to use screening questionnaires either for case finding (i.e. those above the threshold score constitute 'cases' of psychiatric illness) or as a dimension; the full range of scores throughout the population is examined statistically. It is also possible to examine profiles of scores using scaled screening tests, which can also be used as general case detectors by adding the scaled scores together (Goldberg and Williams 1988). For example, the scaled General Health Questionnaire or GHQ-20 was derived by factor analysis and consists of four subscales for somatic symptoms, anxiety and insomnia, social dysfunction and severe depression.

Time frame issues

One limitation of screening tests is deciding what time frame to take for enquiry. If individual items are rated for lifetime ever occurrence (e.g. 'Have you ever had. . . '), it is impossible to know whether the individual items occurred together or at separate times. In disorders such as depression and anxiety, the severity of the psychopathology is related to the number of co-occurring symptoms. Also, most operational definitions of disorder require the co-occurrence of a certain number of symptoms before the diagnosis can be applied. In an attempt to get around this problem, the authors of a self-administered computerized version of CIDI (see chapter 5) defined the time frame very precisely in the questions. Unfortunately this can lead to dense and cumbersome instructions, e.g.:

> For the next few questions please think of the two week period during the
> past 12 months when you had the most complete loss of interest in things.
> During that two week period did the loss of interest usually last . . . (a) all day
> long . . . (b) most of the day . . . (c) about half the day . . . (d) less than half the
> day. (Prince 1998)

An alternative time frame is to use the 'past few weeks' when enquiring about
symptom occurrence. This gets around the need to ask complex questions
about timing of the symptom, as all symptoms that have clustered in the
past few weeks will be acknowledged. However this means that it is only
possible to screen for current psychiatric morbidity, which does lead to
some limitations in applicability. For example lifetime prevalence studies
could not use 'present state' screeners, although they are quite acceptable
for other types of epidemiological research (Prince 1998).

Construction and scoring of screening questionnaires

In screening for multiple, general symptoms, screening questionnaires
have to be broad in their coverage, both in terms of severity and number of items. For example, the original source of items for the GHQ came
from older scales which pre-date modern operational definitions (Goldberg
and Williams 1988). These scales included, the Cornell Medical Inventory
(Brodman *et al.* 1949), McMillan's Health Opinion Survey (McMillan 1959)
and the Gurin Mental Status Index (Gurin *et al.* 1960).

The simplest scoring method is to use a dichotomous, item present or
item absent rating. However, another popular scoring system is to employ a
simple graded approach whereby the subject is given a choice of replies such
as 'mild', 'moderate' or 'severe' in relation to each item. A variation on this is
to ask the subject to quantify how much of the time the symptom has been
present For example a format used in the GHQ is to ask whether a symptom
been present over the past few weeks, 'very often, 'fairly often', 'once in a
while' or 'never'? (Ilfeld 1976). With this method, there are two ways of
calculating scores. A four point response (3, 2, 1 and 0) can be treated
as a *Likert scale* (see chapter 4) and the scores summated over all of the
items. Alternatively, a dichotomous method of scoring can be used where
'very often/fairly often' score one and 'once in a while/never' score zero
(Goldberg 1972). Several other screening and self-report questionnaires

allow the researcher this type of flexibility, but obviously different cut offs for the total scores need to be adopted for each method of scoring (Chalder *et al.* 1993).

Reliability and validity studies of screening questionnaires

The next stage in the development of a screening questionnaire is to undertake reliability and validity studies. Validation of screening questionnaires usually means how well does the screener perform compared to some 'gold standard'. In the past this gold standard was usually a clinician's judgement but, as we discussed in chapter 1, this is also somewhat unreliable. Consequently most modern screening questionnaires have been validated against standardized clinical diagnostic interviews. Again this presupposes that the interview is able to determine 'cases' and 'non cases' of disorder with complete accuracy. The screening questionnaire is then compared with the diagnostic interview in subjects who have been given both. By taking the screener threshold that is assumed to determine caseness, it is then possible to calculate the number of true cases (both screener and interview, positive for caseness), true non-cases (both negative for caseness), false positives (screener positive and interview negative) and false negatives (screener negative and interview positive). It is also straightforward to calculate the *sensitivity* of the screening measure, the proportion of true cases correctly identified, the *specificity* or the proportion of non-cases correctly identified, the *positive predictive value* or the proportion of patients identified as cases that actually are cases according to the criterion and the *negative predictive value,* the proportion of subjects identified as non-cases that are non-cases according to the criterion reference (see also chapter 4).

Increasingly use has been made of receiver (or relative) operating characteristics (ROC) analysis and this has also been described in chapter 4. ROC analysis has the advantage that it allows the screener to be validated across a range of levels of morbidity or for different threshold scores, rather than for just single sensitivity and specificity evaluations.

Screening for psychopathology in primary care

While relatively few individuals attending general practitioner surgeries fulfil operational criteria for mental disorder, significant numbers of general practitioner attendees exhibit some psychiatric morbidity. General practitioners only refer between 10 and 15% of individuals they see with symptoms of mental disorder on to secondary care, and it is estimated that less than 10% of symptomatic individuals see a mental health specialist (Goldberg and Huxley 1992). This means that the majority of those who experience symptoms of mental disorders are managed in primary care.

As well as generally being less severe, the type of psychopathology presenting to general practitioners is somewhat different to that presenting to secondary care services. General practitioners see patients whose complaints do not fit tidily into the diagnostic categories found in traditional psychiatric classifications. For example, complaints such as 'feeling tired all the time', 'needing a tonic', 'feeling worried and anxious', may or may not be pathological (see chapter 1), depending on the precise meaning, associated symptoms, as well as degree of persistence and impairment. Individuals may also visit their general practitioner and discuss relationship problems or social issues such as difficulties with housing. Consequently the 'reason for the visit' may be only indirectly related to mental health. These features of general practice have led to attempts to revise standard classifications and an abbreviated *primary health care* version of the *International Classification of Diseases*, 10th edition, the ICD-10 PHC (WHO 1996, Ustun *et al.* 1995) (and see chapter 5) has undergone field trials in the several countries that have demonstrated the ICD-10 PHC's utility and reliability (Goldberg *et al.* 1995, Goldberg *et al.* 2000).

Screening for psychopathology in medically ill subjects

In-patients in general medical or surgical settings also have high rates of psychopathology; anxiety and depression being commonly associated with being hospitalized. Physical symptoms, such as pain, weight loss and poor sleep are found in both mental and physical illnesses. As in primary care, such individuals do not always fit neatly into the diagnostic categories devised for use by psychiatrists. However, significant impairment and distress may be associated with such symptoms, as well as delay or complications in recovery from the physical illness, and if identified such symptoms can be often be treated. Screening for psychopathology in such groups has specific requirements; for example individuals may be physically unable to write, or pain may limit concentration and the ability to complete lengthy questionnaires. Although less severely and acutely ill, those attending outpatient clinics (called 'ambulatory' patients in the US) also have higher rates of depressive and anxiety symptoms compared to the general population. As well as the GHQ, a number of other self-report screening questionnaires have been used with such patient groups (see table 7.1)

Some of the commonly used screening questionnaires

The General Health Questionnaire (GHQ)

The GHQ is one of the best known and commonly used screening questionnaires for general psychopathology. Originally devised to detect psychiatric morbidity in the general population in the UK (Goldberg 1972), the GHQ has been translated into 38 languages and over 50 validity studies have been published (Goldberg and Williams 1988). The GHQ has also been used extensively in primary care settings. It focuses on the main common types of psychopathology; depression, anxiety, and somatic concerns (Goldberg 1972), in particular measuring recent change in psychological functioning. An early version of the GHQ consisted of 140 items, but after extensive testing in different groups of subjects, both with and without mental disorder, as well as further statistical refinement, the 60-item GHQ (GHQ-60) was finally published in 1972 (Goldberg 1972). Further research over the years has led to the development of even shorter versions, the shortest of which is the 12-item GHQ (Goldberg and Williams 1988).

For several decades, the GHQ has been used to screen for psychiatric disorder in primary care (Goldberg and Huxley 1992). Many studies in the UK and internationally, confirm that the GHQ is both valid and reliable in such settings (Lee *et al.* 1997).

The Beck Depression Inventory (BDI)

According to Richter and colleagues (1998) in over 2,000 empirical studies, the BDI (Beck 1961) is one of the most used self-report questionnaires for depression. Despite some shortcomings, e.g. high item difficulty, lack of representative norms, controversial factorial validity, and poor discriminant validity against anxiety, the questionnaire has considerable advantages e.g. high internal consistency and content validity as well as validity in differentiating depressed from non depressed subjects (Richter *et al.* 1998). The BDI has been used to measure change in depressive symptoms over time.

Table 7.1. Some questionnaires used to screen for psychopathology and to rate change.

Name	Author (s)	Application	Symptoms covered
General Health Questionnaire (GHQ)	Goldberg 1972	Primary care, general population and hospital settings	Depression, anxiety and somatic symptoms
Beck Depression Inventory (BDI)*	Beck et al. 1961	Epidemiological and general hospital settings	Depression and anxiety symptoms
Zung scales	Zung 1990	Primary care, medically ill, low functioning subjects	Separate scales for depression and anxiety. Interviewer-assisted version
Psychiatric Symptom Index (PSI)	Ilfield 1976	General population	Depression and anxiety symptoms
Center for Epidemiological Studies Depression Scale (CES-D)*	Radloff 1977	Epidemiological settings	Depressive symptoms. Automated telephone versions
Primary Care Evaluation of Mental disorders (PRIME-MD)	Spitzer et al. 1994	Primary care	Rapid screen of general psychiatric morbidity
Symptom Driven Diagnostic System for Primary Care (SDDS-PC)	Broadbent et al. 1995	Primary care	General psychiatric morbidity (DSMIV); includes screener of functional impairment
Association for Methodology and Documentation in Psychiatry (AMDP)	Pietzcker and Gebhardt 1983	Psychiatric patients	Psychopathological somatic and anamnestic symptoms

Table 7.1. (cont.)

Name	Author (s)	Application	Symptoms covered
Hamilton Rating Scales: (HAM-D, HAS, IRS HADS and CRS)*	Hamilton 1960 (and other authors – see text)	Psychiatric patients	Depression and anxiety (observer and self-rated versions)
Brief Psychiatric Rating Scale (BPRS)*	Overall and Gorham 1962	Psychiatric patients	General psychiatric symptoms, mainly psychosis
Scales for assessment of positive and negative symptoms (SANS, SAPS and PANNS)*	Andreasen and Olsen 1982 Kay et al. 1987	Subjects with schizophrenia	Symptoms and subtypes of schizophrenia
Comprehensive psychopathological Rating Scale (CPRS)* and Montgomery-Asberg Depression Rating Scale (MADRS)*	Asberg and Shalling 1979 Montgomery and Asberg 1979	Psychiatric patients	CPRS: subscales for different syndromes MADRS: depression (observer rated)

Key to abbreviations:
HAM-D Hamilton Depression Rating Scale
HAS Hamilton Anxiety Scale
IRS Irritability Rating Scale
HADS Hospital Anxiety and Depression Rating Scale
CRS Carroll Rating Scale

There is also ample evidence that it can be used effectively for screening in epidemiological, primary care and general hospital settings (Lasa *et al.* 2000, Winter *et al.* 1999, Lykouras *et al.* 1998, Beck *et al.* 1997).

The Zung Scales

The Zung self report depression scale (SDS) and Zung self report anxiety scale (SAS) have been also been used widely in primary care (Zung 1990), with medically ill subjects, and in those with alcohol problems (Lippman *et al.* 1987). The Zung SDS has also been shown to have cross cultural applicability (Fugita and Crittenden 1990) and to be a valid screen for depression in the elderly (DeForge and Sobal 1988) including those with low severity Alzheimer's dementia (Gottlieb *et al.* 1988). The questionnaire can be orally presented to low functioning psychiatric patients with good reliability (Griffin and Kogout 1988), and a short interviewer-assisted version has also been shown to work well with elderly subjects (Tucker *et al.* 1987).

Psychiatric Symptom Index (PSI)

The PSI is a shortened version of the Hopkins Symptom Distress Checklist (Parloff *et al.* 1954) constructed for a general population study of stress and coping (Ilfeld 1976). It consists of twenty-nine items relating to depression and anxiety, and has been shown to have stable psychometric properties in several US populations (Stein and Jessop 1989). It has also been shown (Bauman 1994) that a total score on PSI greater than thirty indicates a high likelihood of a diagnosis of major depression on the Diagnostic Interview Schedule (DIS – see chapter 3) (Robins *et al.* 1981). More recently, a content analysis against DSM-IV criteria for depression and anxiety has supported the applicability of the scale for current research (Okun *et al.* 1996).

Center for Epidemiological Studies-Depression Scale

The twenty items that make up this screening questionnaire for depressive symptoms, were originally included in a lengthy structured interview used in a large epidemiological study undertaken in the Midwest of the USA between 1971 and 1973 (Radloff 1977). The CES-D has been shown to be a sensitive tool for detecting depressive symptoms in psychiatric populations and change of symptoms over time (Weissman *et al.* 1977). When completing the CES-D, the subject is asked to use a four-point scale to respond to twenty items relating to 'the past week' (Okun *et al.* 1996). The CES-D has been validated in different countries, and translated into different languages including Arabic and Chinese (Ghubash *et al.* 2000). In addition, the scale has recently been administered in two interview formats in English and Spanish; a speech recognition program presented by cellular telephone and a face-to-face method (Munoz *et al.* 1999). The authors concluded that the automated version of the CES-D was acceptable and valid in both Spanish and English speakers.

The Primary Care Evaluation of Mental Disorders (PRIME-MD)

This short interview has been devised to provide a rapid diagnostic procedure for primary care physicians in the US. Based on DSM-IIIR operational criteria, the approximately 8 minute assessment has been shown to have good diagnostic agreement with independent mental health professionals (Spitzer *et al.* 1994). However, 8 minutes of professional time is too long for primary care physicians, so the authors have recently introduced a modified self-report version, the Patient Health Questionnaire (PHQ) (Spitzer *et al.* 1999). In addition, a computerized self-administered version of PRIME-MD was found to acceptable to emergency department attendees who completed the questionnaire in a median time of 7 minutes (Schriger *et al.* 2001). However, although 42% of subjects received a PRIME-MD diagnosis, their physicians rarely diagnosed or treated these conditions, even when given these diagnoses.

The Symptom Driven Diagnostic System for Primary Care (SDDS-PC)

Another recent screen test, also devised to find cases defined according to American Psychiatric Association DSMIIIR criteria, is the Symptom-Driven Diagnostic System for Primary Care (SDDS-PC) (Broadhead *et al.* 1995). The original 62 items relating to 9 mental disorders was reduced to 16, following analysis of item and scale performance. The self-administered SDDS-PC provides a 'sensitive, valid and patient friendly first step' to the recognition and management of mental disorders in primary care that, according to the authors, also aids the physician in the selection of appropriate diagnostic interview modules for the disorders that screened positive (Broadbent *et al.* 1995). The screener also include the examination of functional impairment (Leon *et al.* 1996).

The Association for Methodology and Documentation in Psychiatry (AMDP) system and scales

Founded by a group of German, Austrian and Swiss psychiatrists in 1965, the Association for Methodology and Documentation in Psychiatry (AMDP) developed a uniform and comprehensive system for documenting psychopathological, somatic and amnestic symptoms. The AMDP syndrome scales were based on analyses of the symptoms presented by mentally ill subjects attending the psychiatric clinics in Munich, Zurich and later Berlin (Pietzcker and Gebhardt 1983). In 1981, a revision of the scales was undertaken following the evaluation of data from French and Belgian subjects (Bobon *et al.* 1982), and standardization against the Research Diagnostic Criteria was undertaken a year or two later (Doumont *et al.* 1982, Ansseau *et al.* 1982).

Rating scales devised to measure change in severity of psychopathology

The need to measure change in treatment trials has generated a demand for valid, reliable questionnaires that can measure change in severity of psychopathology over time. By far the greatest area of attention has been on evaluating depressive symptomology, and to a lesser extent, anxiety, although we shall also discuss three important scales used to measure change in the symptoms of schizophrenia. While many are self-report, some are observer, clinician or nurse rating questionnaires. As with screening questionnaires, their use has broadened over time, with the best-known questionnaires having been used in various research settings.

As with screening questionnaires, issues regarding validity and reliability have to be addressed and the psychometric properties of the questionnaire determined. The older questionnaires were validated against 'expert' clinical judgement (Snaith 1996) whilst for those devised more recently, diagnoses derived from structured diagnostic interviews or older questionnaires have been used as validating criterion measures.

Self report versus observer rated questionnaires

Both self-report and observer rating scales have advantages and disadvantages. As we have noted above, self-rating scales are quick and cheap to administer, and may even be sent via the post to be completed. Observer rated scales require the raters to be trained, and inter-rater reliability must be acceptable (see chapter 4). Such scales are generally considered to be inherently more conservative when compared to self-report scales. However, Edwards and colleagues comparison study of the BDI and Hamilton Rating Scale for Depression (HAM-D) cast some doubts on this assumption, as they found that the self-report BDI was more conservative than the observer rated HAM-D (Edwards *et al.* 1984). Feinberg and colleagues (1981) compared four depression rating scales; two observer rated and two self-report, (the HAM-D, the Clinical Global Rating of Depression, a visual analogue scale (see chapter 4), and the Carroll Rating Scale respectively) in depressed subjects attending an outpatient clinic. These authors showed that the overall correlations between the two self rated and two observer rated scales were highly significant, and that there was little advantage of one type of scale over the other. However, there is a tendency for some groups of depressed subjects to self-report their symptoms as more severe than a clinical observer.

Some of the more popular scales devised to rate change in severity

The Hamilton Rating Scales

One of the earliest depression rating scales to be devised and still one of the most widely used in treatment trials is the Hamilton Depression Rating Scale (HAM-D) (Hamilton 1960). Although this scale is forty years old, it is still used in a way that is close to its original format. In a recent study of research practise, Snaith (1996) examined the method for evaluating depression in articles published in five leading psychiatric journals and found that 66% of the sventy-five papers that had used a standard measure of depression had used the HAM-D. Originally consisting of seventeen items, each rated for severity on a two or three-point scale, the HAM-D was devised to assess symptom severity in subjects with a clinical diagnosis of depression (Hamilton 1960, 1967). The author recommended that the scale should be completed by two independent raters, employing information derived from all available sources, including ward nurses and family informants as well as from interviews with the depressed subject (Hamilton 1960, Snaith 1996). However not all of those who have used the scale have followed these requirements (Snaith 1996). Subsequently, the author added a further four items (21-item version) (Hamilton 1967). The HAM-D has been shown to have high correlation scores when compared with psychiatrist's global rating (Knesevich *et al.* 1977) and to discriminate effectively between normal subjects and those with depression (Fava *et al.* 1982). However there have been critics of the scale, in respect of poor internal consistency (Bech and Coppen 1990) and a lack of explicit guidance for the severity ratings (Bech and Coppen 1990). As a result of these perceived shortcomings in the HAM-D, the 1970s and 1980s saw a proliferation in the publication of alternative rating scales for measuring change in severity of depressive and anxiety symptoms (Maier *et al.* 1988, Guelfi 1988, Asberg and Schalling 1979, Woggon 1979, Carroll *et al.* 1981).

Around the same time as the HAM-D was being constructed Hamilton (1959) also devised a scale to evaluate 'neurotic anxiety'. Subsequently Hamilton's colleagues produced other scales to rate irritability, depression and anxiety (Snaith *et al.* 1978), and a self- report scale designed to be used with hospital patients including the medically ill, the Hospital Anxiety and Depression Scale (HADS) (Zigmond and Snaith 1983).

Also at the beginning of the 1980s, the Carroll Rating Scale (CRS) was developed to be a self rather than observer rating scale. The information content and specific items of the CRS closely match the HAM-D (Carroll *et al.* 1981) and the CRS and HAM-D have been shown to have correlate well (Carroll *et al.* 1981, Nasr *et al.* 1984).

The Brief Psychiatric Rating Scale (BPRS)

Also dating from the early 1960s, the Brief Psychiatric Rating Scale (Overall and Gorham 1962) is still used to assess efficacy in psychopharmacological research, mainly in relation to psychotic symptoms (Noordsy *et al.* 2001). The scale consists of eighteen symptom constructs that are rated on a seven point severity scale. However, like the HAM-D, the lack of cues for rating severity caused misgivings about the consistency of ratings across different centres (Manchander *et al.* 1989). To overcome this criticism, an 'anchored' version (i.e. with cues provided for severity rating), the BPRS-A, has been produced that has been shown to be of use clinically in facilitating the differential diagnosis of in-patients (Hopko *et al.* 2001). Also a children's version, the BPRS-C, has also been developed (Hughes *et al.* 2001).

Scale for the Assessment of Positive Symptoms (SAPS) and Scale for the Assessment of Negative Symptoms (SANS) and the Positive and Negative Symptom Scales (PANSS)

The SANS and SAPS rating scales for schizophrenia (Andreasen and Olsen 1982) were devised on the basis of the observation that certain symptom profiles appeared to be related to cerebral ventricular size as measured on computerized tomography (CT) scans (Andreasen *et al.* 1982). The authors noted that large ventricles and cognitive impairment were related to a preponderance of negative symptoms such as poverty of speech, lack of motivation, affective flattening and anhedonia (see chapter 2). On the other hand, small ventricles corresponded to an excess of 'positive' symptoms such as delusions and hallucinations (Andreasen *et al.* 1982). Although the scales allow schizophrenia to be sub-typed into positive and negative categories (Andreasen *et al.* 1990), SAPS and SANS have mainly been used a dimensional scales to rate change over time, particularly in drug trials. Most drug treatments for schizophrenia lead to the improvement of positive, rather than negative symptoms. Consequently, there has been much research activity to find more effective treatment for negative symptoms.

The 30-item PANSS scale (Kay *et al.* 1987) was based on the earlier SAPS and SANS scales. The authors stated that PANSS was designed as 'an operationalized, drug-sensitive instrument' providing a 'balanced representation of positive and negative symptoms', their 'relationship to one another, and to global psychopathology' (Kay *et al.* 1987). The PANSS scale continues to be widely used as a dimensional measure of symptom change in schizophrenia research including treatment outcome, quality of life, neuroimaging and cognitive studies (Black *et al.* 2001, Brebion *et al.* 2001).

The Comprehensive Psychopathological Rating Scale (CPRS) and the Montgomery-Asberg Depression Rating Scale (MADRS)

The CPRS, devised in Sweden, consists of sixty-five scaled items covering a wide range of psychiatric symptoms, with explicit definitions for each item as well as the scaled steps (Asberg and Schalling 1979). The CPRS and related scales have been devised to measure treatment effects. The scale is rated via an interview, and can be used in full or as a pool of items to devise subscales for different psychiatric syndromes. The CPRS has been shown to have good reliability and validity, and can be applied by those from different training backgrounds, including social workers and nurses (Perris 1979).

The 10-item Montgomery-Asberg Depression Rating Scale (MADRS) (Montgomery and Asberg 1979) was devised from the items of the CPRS depression subscale. Another ten CPRS items relating to anxiety symptoms have been brought together to provide a 'brief scale for anxiety'(Tyrer *et al.* 1984). An extended version of the CPRS depression subscale plus some additional items has also been shown to differentiate between ill and recovered as well as bipolar patients (Perris *et al.* 1984).

In this chapter, we have described some of the more commonly used ratings scales that are used to screen for psychopathology and or to rate change in severity of symptoms. In chapter 8 we will continue with the theme of ratings scales, but will present those used in special groups, such as the elderly or children or with specific disorders such as substance misuse.

Measuring Psychopathology in Specific Subject Groups

Introduction

Measuring psychopathology in particular groups of subjects may require diagnostic assessments, instruments or rating scales that are tailor made to their requirements. Such subjects include children and adolescents, those with a learning disability (mental retardation), and the elderly, especially those who are cognitively impaired. Self-expression and awareness may be limited in these groups and so observer information assumes greater importance than in subjects who can give a more detailed self-report. Also the mental health problems, syndromes and disorders experienced by these

Table 8.1. Features of depression in children compared
with adults (Hill 1997).

Common presentations in children	Common presentations in adults
Social withdrawal	Delusions
Irritability	Suicide
Running away from home	Altered libido
Separation anxiety	Sleep disturbance
Pain in head, chest, or abdomen	Weight loss
Decline in school work	

three subject groups can be somewhat different to those we have already discussed in relation to non-intellectually impaired adults. For example, while the presentation of obsessive-compulsive disorder is similar in children and adults, the clinical features of depression are rather different in these two age groups (see table 8.1) (Hill 1997).

In addition, disturbances of behaviour or conduct are much more prominent, not only in children but also in those with learning disability and the elderly mentally ill. Distress due to pain or emotional problems may be expressed via changes in behaviour rather than verbally. Developmental issues, socializing and scholastic ability are important considerations in children and adolescents, while intellectual ability or decline influence the measurement of psychopathology in the learning disabled and elderly. In this chapter we will review the diagnostic interviews and rating scales that are used in these subject groups.

Other 'special groups' in respect of measuring psychopathology are those who misuse street drugs and/or alcohol, those who have eating disorders and those who have just given birth. Mind altering drugs (including alcohol) and the impact of starvation can both alter the nature and presentation of psychopathology. Similarly, childbirth is associated with excess rates of mental disorder, mainly depression. We will also discuss some of the interviews and ratings scales devised to evaluate specific types of psychopathology associated with these subject groups.

Classification of psychopathology in children and adolescents

The background to the development of a nosology for this age group parallels that of adults. In Europe, childhood psychiatric disorder was defined according to the ideas of impairment, suffering or abnormalities of development (Hill 1997). In North America, the prominence of the psychoanalytic movement has influenced the definition of disorder. However, as in adults, disorders affecting children and adolescents are now defined operationally (see chapter 3 and table 3.1), and there is much improved diagnostic reliability, and international agreement. Indeed, both DSMIV and ICD10 have specific codes and sections covering the disorders presenting in childhood and adolescence (see table 8.2). In addition, there is also an ongoing debate about the need to employ a dimensional approach as well as categorical definitions of disorder (Achenbach and Edelbrock 1978, Plomin *et al.* 1991).

Table 8.2. ICD10 main diagnostic groups for disorders of childhood and adolescence.

F70–79 Mental retardation
  F70 Mild mental retardation
  F71 Moderate mental retardation
  F72 Severe mental retardation
  F73 Profound mental retardation

Fourth character denotes extent of associated behavioural impairment

F80–89 Disorders of psychological development
  F80 Specific developmental disorder of speech and language, e.g. specific speech articulation disorder (stammering)
  F81 Specific developmental disorder of scholastic skills. e.g. dyslexia, dyscalculia
  F82 Specific developmental disorder of motor function
  F84 Pervasive developmental disorders, e.g. childhood autism, Rett's syndrome, Asperger's syndrome

F90–99 Behavioural and emotional disorders with onset usually occurring in childhood and adolescence
  F90 Hyperkinetic disorders, e.g. ADHD
  F91 Conduct disorders, e.g. oppositional defiant disorder (temper tantrums)
  F93 Emotional disorders with onset specific to childhood, e.g. separation anxiety disorder (school phobia)
  F94 Disorders of social functioning with onset specific to childhood, e.g. elective mutism (choosing not to speak)
  F98 Other behavioural and emotional disorders with onset usually occurring in childhood and adolescence, e.g. eneuresis, encopresis (incontinence of urine and faeces, respectively)

Both ICD10 and DSMIV employ a multi-axial classification for disorders found in children and adolescents. For ICD10 the axes are:

- Axis I, clinical psychiatric syndromes
- Axis II specific disorders of development
- Axis III intellectual level
- Axis IV associated medical conditions
- Axis V associated abnormal psychosocial conditions, and
- Axis VI global social functioning.

In DSMIV, the same axial framework for adults is applied to children and adolescents (see chapter 3).

Diagnostic interviews and rating scales used with children and adolescents

For older children and adolescents it is possible to carry out interviews with the young person themselves (Hodges 1993), while for younger children it is generally either the parent or a teacher who is asked about the child's psychopathology. Below the age of 9, children are unreliable informants of the timing, onset, duration and severity of symptoms, although they can describe moods, feelings and some antisocial activities, such as lying or stealing (Angold 2000). A number of structured and semi-structured interviews have been designed for use with older children, parents and teachers, and these are shown in table 8.3.

All the interviews listed in table 8.3 show considerable overlap, although two broad types of interview emerge. All cover the diagnostic categories included in the most recent operational definitions for childhood disorders, namely DSMIIIR, DSMIV, and ICD10, although some are mainly devised for epidemiological use, and therefore can be given by lay interviewers, while others are mainly for use in a clinical setting and require clinicians to be the interviewers. In these respects the approach to measuring psychopathology resembles that for adults, in that the items required to fulfil the operational criteria for each diagnosis are formulated into a question, or series of questions, to be asked by the interviewer. Computerized scoring programs can then be used or hand-scoring algorithms applied so that 'a diagnosis' can be assigned.

The main interviews used in this age range are, the Child and Adolescent Psychiatric Assessment (CAPA) (Angold *et al.* 1995), the Schedules for Affective Disorders and Schizophrenia for school-aged children (K-SADS) (Chambers *et al.* 1985), the Diagnostic Interview for Children and Adolescents (DICA) (Welner *et al.* 1987), the Diagnostic Interview for Children (DISC) (Costello *et al.* 1985) and the Child Assessment Schedule (CAS) (Hodges *et al.* 1982). More recently, a childhood disorders version of the SCID (see chapter 5), the Structured Clinical Interview for DSMIV Childhood Disorders (KID-SCID) has also been made available (Matzner *et al.* 1997).

The Child and Adolescent Psychiatric Assessment (CAPA) (Angold *et al.* 1994) is a semi-structured investigator-based schedule that can be used with parents or children over the age of 8 years. The interview covers all psychiatric morbidity found children and adolescents, with the exception of developmental disorders.

The Schedule for Affective Disorders and Schizophrenia for school-aged children (K-SADS) (Chambers *et al.* 1985) is a version of the adult SADS (see chapter 5) designed for use with children. While the interview is comprehensive in its coverage of psychiatric morbidity, its original application was the evaluation of the present mental state. However, subsequent versions, compatible with the DSMIV classification (American Psychiatric Association 1994) have been published including a 'present state' and 'lifetime ever', (the K-SADS-PL, and the K-SADS-E,) both intended for epidemiological use (Kaufman *et al.* 1997, Ambrosini 2000).

Similarly the Diagnostic Interview for Children and Adolescents (DICA) (Welner *et al.* 1987) has been designed along similar lines to an adult interview, namely the DIS (see chapter 5). DICA has been specifically designed for use by lay interviewers, and its original format was highly structured. However a revised version is semi-structured, and can be given to young children (Reich 2000). Three computerized versions of the interview are also available for different age groups (Reich *et al.* 1995).

Also following the trend of producing child versions of adult interviews, the KID-SCID was developed in 1993, although reliability and validity data was not presented for the interview until 1997 (Matzner 1997). Designed as a semi-structured instrument for clinical research use, the authors maintain that KID-SCID is easy to use, has utility as a training tool and has excellent inter-rater reliability (Matzner 1997).

Table 8.3. Interviews to evaluate psychopathology in children and adolescents (C and A).

Name	Author(s)	Type of interview	What is measured	Age range	Time to administer	Training required
The Child and Adolescent Psychiatric Assessment (CAPA)	Angold et al. 1995	Semi-structured	All C and A psychiatric disorders except developmental disorders	8–16 (Child) 4–16 (Parent)	Around 2 hours	Yes
Schedule for Affective Disorders and Schizophrenia for school aged children(K-SADS)	Chambers et al. 1985 Ambrosini 2000	Semi-structured (based on adult interview SADS) Clinicians should administer	All C and A psychiatric disorders	Not specified	Not specified	Not specified
Diagnostic interview for children and adolescent (DICA) plus revised version (DICA-R)	Welner et al. 1987 Reich 2000	Highly structured can be used by lay interviewer	All C and A psychiatric disorders	Not specified	Not specified	Yes
Structured Clinical Interview for DSMIV Childhood Diagnoses (KID-SCID)	Matzner 1997	Semi-structured based on adult interview SCID. Clinicians should administer	All C and A psychiatric disorders	Not specified	—	—

Table 8.3. (*Continued*)

Name	Author(s)	Type of interview	What is measured	Age range	Time to administer	Training required
Diagnostic interview for children (DISC) and revised version (DISC-R)	Costello *et al.* 1985 Shaffer *et al.* 1993	Highly structured can be used by lay interviewer specifically developed for epidemiological use	All C and A psychiatric disorders	Not specified	Not specified	Yes
Child Assessment Schedule (CAS)	Hodges *et al.* 1982	Semi-structured clinical interview based on around thematic topics (school, friend, family etc).	All C and A psychiatric disorders	Not specified	Not specified	Not specified

The Diagnostic Interview Schedule for Children (DISC) (Costello *et al.* 1985) was also originally designed for use by lay interviewers in epidemiological studies. A revised version improved some unreliable and undiscriminating items (Shaffer *et al.* 1993). Version 2.1C of DISC has also been shown to have reasonable re-test stability in Anglo, African and Hispanic adolescents (Roberts *et al.* 1996).

The Child Assessment Schedule (CAS) is a longer semi-structured, thematically organized interview for use by clinicians, and is one of the older diagnostic interviews used in this age range (Hodges *et al.* 1982). In a comparative study of parents and childrens' accounts of behavioural and emotional problems using the CAS, Verhulst and colleagues (1987) found relatively high agreement, although parents tended to score higher for their children's symptoms than the children themselves, with the exception of fears and anxiety, where the children scored higher.

Self-report and Screening Questionnaires

These 'pencil and paper tests', are designed to be completed by the subjects themselves in the case of older children or adolescents, or by non-clinician observers, most commonly parents or teachers or both. They mainly require no training, and are generally completed in a few minutes. While some take a broad brief and cover the main conduct and emotional disorders of childhood, others are more specific and are focused on particular groups of symptoms such as those of anxiety, depression or hyperactivity. Some have been designed primarily for screening or epidemiological research. Since the child's stage of development and age are important correlates to the evaluation of psychopathology, scales such the Vineland Adaptive Behaviour Scale (Sparrow *et al.* 1984) provides measures of the achievement of developmental *milestones* (i.e. the ages at which children talk, play with peers, read etc).

Some of the more widely used self-report, screening, parent and teacher questionnaires used to evaluate psychopathology in children and adolescents are shown in table 8.4. General purpose screening questionnaires are the Rutter scales (Rutter *et al.* 1975) and the Strengths and Difficulties Questionnaire (Goodman 1997) and the Ontario Child Health Study Scales (Boyle *et al.* 1993). The Child Behaviour Checklist (CBCL) (Achenbach and Edelbrock 1978) provides a comprehensive checklist of behavioural and social competences covering 2–18 years. More specific questionnaires include the Conners parent and teacher rating scales for attention deficit hyperactivity disorder (ADHD) and the Olwens scales for conduct disorders (Conners 1998, Olwens 1993). Depression and anxiety disorders in childhood can be screened for using the Child Depression Inventory (CDI) (Kovacs 1981), a childhood version of the Beck Depression Inventory (see chapter 7) or the Moods and Feelings Questionnaire (Costello and Angold 1985). The 'What I think and feel' questionnaire (Reynolds and Richmond 1997) provides a screener for anxiety disorders. Specific scales for autistic spectrum disorders include the Autism Behavioural Checklist (Nordin and Gillberg 1996), the Real Life Rating Scale (Freeman *et al.* 1986) and the Childhood Autism Rating Scale (Schopler *et al.* 1980).

Evaluating psychopathology in those with learning disability (mental retardation)

The last three decades have been described as the 'age of enlightenment' for individuals with intellectual impairment (Fraser 2000). As well as major advances in knowledge, there has also been a transformation in service provision. However these changes have been associated with confusion over terminology. The UK government dispensed with the stigmatizing term 'mentally handicapped' in 1990, and substituted 'learning disabled' to those individuals who, according to DSMIV criteria, have 'sub-average general intelligence' (i.e. an Intelligence Quotient or IQ of less than 70). However the American Association of Mental Retardation has retained the term 'mental retardation' because it is less confusing and is better recognized internationally. This terminology is also congruent with the definitions included in the *International Classification of Impairments, Disabilities and Handicaps* (WHO 1980). However, irrespective of the 'label' that is applied, what such individuals have in common is significant intellectual impairment that is associated with difficulty in acquiring basic living, educational and social skills (Holland 2000).

DSMIV defines 'mental retardation' according to four categories, (mild, moderate severe and profound) on the basis of IQ score (see also table 8.2 for ICD10 categories). Clearly, the established tests of intellectual function such as the Wechsler Adult Intelligence Test (WAIS) (Wechsler 1997) and the Wechsler Intelligence Tests for Children (WISC) (Wechsler 1992) have a key role defining the basic level of 'impairment'. However individuals

Table 8.4. Some self-report, screening and parent and teachers questionnaires used to evaluate psychopathology in children and adolescents.

Type	Name	Authors	Comments
General purpose Screening questionnaires	Rutter parents (A2) and teachers (B2) scales	Rutter et al. 1975	Widely used and many translations. Preschool and prosocial versions also available.
	Strengths and Difficulties Questionnaires	Goodman 1997	Based on Rutter and Prosocial Behavioural Scales. Completed by parents and teachers
	Ontario Child Health Study Scales	Boyle et al. 1993	Devised for epidemiological study of child mental health in Ontario. Comprehensive set of scales with good reliability and validity
Comprehensive checklist	Child Behaviour Check List (CBCL)	Achenbach and Edelbrock 1978	30–45 minutes to complete. Covers behavioural and social competence over 6 months for 2–18 year olds

Table 8.4. (*Continued*)

Type	Name	Authors	Comments
Behavioural problems including Attention Deficit Hyperactivity Disorder (ADHD)	Conners parent and teacher rating scales revised	Conners 1998	Screening questionnaires for ADHD. Also used to monitor treatment response
Assessment of depression and anxiety	Child Depression Inventory	Kovacs 1981	Based on Beck Depression Inventory
	Moods & Feelings Questionnaire	Costello and Angold 1985	Can be administered in groups, individually or sent via mail
	What I think & Feel	Reynolds and Richmond 1997	Screens for anxiety disorders
Assessment of Conduct disorders	Olwens Scales	Olwens 1993	Screens for conduct disorders
Development and adaptive functioning	Vineland Adaptive Behaviour Scales	Sparrow *et al.* 1984	Provides normal 'developmental milestones'
Pervasive development disorder	Autistic Behavioural Check List	Nordin Gillberg 1996 Freeman *et al.* 1986	Scales for autistic spectrum disorders
	Real Life Rating Scale		
	Childhood Autism Rating Scale	Schopler *et al.* 1980	

with mental retardation don't only have impairment. They usually also have 'disability' and/or 'handicap', neither, of which can be evaluated by the application of IQ tests alone. Disability has been defined by the WHO (1980) as a 'restriction or lack of ability to perform an activity in a manner or within the range considered normal for a human being'. Scales such as the Vineland Adaptive Behavior Scales (Sparrow *et al.* 1984), and the American Adaptive Behavior Scales (Nihara *et al.* 1993) can be used to assess disability. Similarly, 'handicap' has been defined by the WHO (1980) as 'a disadvantage for a given individual resulting from an impairment or disability that limits or prevents the fulfilment of a role that is normal for that individual'. 'Quality of life' measures (Lehman 1996, Wiersma 1996) (and see also chapter 10) can be applied to the evaluation of handicap. Recently the learning disability faculty of the Royal College of Psychiatrists in the UK has published a detailed interpretation of the ICD 10 criteria that assists the clinician in applying the various components of the classification (Royal College of Psychiatrists 2001).

Individuals with mental retardation can suffer from the same range of mental disorders as those with normal intellectual abilities. Indeed, severe psychiatric disorder is two to three times more common in those with mental retardation than in the non-intellectually impaired (Einfield and Tonge 1996). However, assessment methods have to be modified for those with limited ability to describe their mental life, and to take into account indirect evidence for psychopathology on the basis of carers' reports. For example, depression may be expressed by tearfulness, irritability and lack of appetite or sleep that may be observed by a carer, rather than complained of by the subject. Similarly, odd behaviour, rather than verbal descriptions of the 'voices', may imply the presence of hallucinations. However, structured mental state assessment instruments are available such as the Psychopathology Instrument for Mentally Retarded Adults (Matson *et al.* 1984) and the Psychiatric Assessment for Adults with Developmental Disorders (PAS-ADD) (Moss 1993). Also there are sections in the SCAN interview, (see chapter 5) that deal with disorders associated with developmental delay, such as autistic spectrum disorders and Asberger's syndrome (Wing *et al.* 1990).

There are also a number of rating scales and neuropsychological tests that can be effectively used with subjects who have intellectual impairment. Dementia can develop in the elderly mentally impaired just as in those whose intellectual abilities are within the normal range, although the early stages of the disorder may present somewhat differently (Aylward *et al.* 1997). In a recent comparison study of three different questionnaires and scales with clinical diagnosis, Deb and Braganza (1999) concluded that observer rated scales (i.e. the Dementia Scale for Persons with Mental Retardation and the Dementia Scale for Down's Syndrome) performed better than direct neuropsychological tests (i.e. the Mini Mental State Examination) in diagnosing dementia in those with intellectual impairment.

As mentioned in the introduction to this chapter, those with mental retardation may also have behavioural disturbances, sometimes also called 'challenging behaviour'. This may occur in relation to physical health problems such as epilepsy, which are more common in those with mental retardation than the general population. Alternatively, challenging behaviour may be an indication of the presence of psychopathology. Disruptive and aggressive behaviour is more commonly associated with milder retardation, while those with severe disability are more likely to be withdrawn and autistic. Tonge and colleagues (1996) have described the use of factor analysis to ascertain patterns of psychopathology in children with mental retardation. The authors examined six commonly used rating scales and found six fairly consistent groupings of disturbance. These were aggression-antisocial behaviour, social withdrawal, stereotypic behaviours, hyperactive disruptive behaviours, repetitive communication disturbance and anxiety fearfulness (Tonge *et al.* 1996). Two questionnaires that cover these six types of disturbance have been specifically designed and validated for children with mental retardation. They are the Developmental Behaviour Checklist (Einfeld and Tonge 1992) and the Nisonger Child Behaviour Rating Form (Aman *et al.* 1996).

Measuring psychopathology and cognitive decline in the elderly

Cognitive decline and impairment can also lead to modifications in the presentation of psychopathology. In many respects these are similar to those outlined above in relation to learning disability, where carers may be better informants that the subjects themselves. Behavioural disturbance or irritability may be the only indications of depression or psychosis. Similarly, depression can cause a false picture of dementia (pseudo-dementia) in this age group. Consequently evaluation of cognitive status is a central part of the examination for psychopathology in the elderly.

Table 8.5. Interviews and rating scales used in those with learning disability (mental retardation)

Name	Author(s)	What is measured
Wechsler Adult Intelligence Scale (WAIS)	Wechsler 1997	IQ impairment
Wechsler Intelligence Scales for Children (WISC)	Wechsler 1992	IQ impairment
Vineland Adaptive Behavior Scales	Sparrow *et al.* 1984	Disability
American Adaptive Behavior Scales	Nihara *et al.* 1993	Disability
Psychopathology Instrument for Mentally Retarded Adults	Matson *et al.* 1984	General psychopathology
Psychiatric Assessment for Adults with Developmental Disorders (PAS-ADD)	Moss 1993	General psychopathology
Schedules for the Clinical Assessment of Neuropsychiatry(SCAN)	Wing *et al.* 1990	Autistic spectrum disorders, dementia
Dementia Scale for Persons with Mental Retardation	Hooge Burch 1992	Dementia
Dementia Scale for Down's Syndrome	Huxley *et al.* 2000	Dementia
Developmental Behaviour Checklist	Einfield and Tonge 1992	Challenging behaviour
Nisonger Child Behaviour Rating Form	Aman *et al.* 1996	Challenging behaviour

The Cambridge Mental Disorders of the Elderly Examination (CAMDEX) is a good example of a widely used diagnostic instrument, appropriate for clinical and research application (Roth *et al.* 1986). It consists of three components; the first is a structured clinical interview with the patient, concerning their present physical and mental state, activities of daily living, past and family history and a physical examination including a neurological assessment. The second focuses on the same issues but comprises a structured interview with a relative or other informant able to provide independent information. The third component consists of a cognitive examination and is called the CAMCOG. The CAMCOG incorporates items from the Mini-Mental State Examination (MMSE), tests a broad range of cognitive processes and provides a detailed measure of memory processes, assessing orientation, language, memory, praxis, attention, abstract thinking, perception and calculation. Following the CAMDEX interview, the interviewer also records observations on the patient's appearance, behaviour, mood, speech, mental slowing, activity, insight, thought processes and level of consciousness and any bizarre behaviour observed. The whole assessment process is estimated to take 1 hour and 20 minutes.

Roth and colleagues (1986) report evidence of good inter-rater reliability and of significant agreement between subsections of the scales incorporated in CAMDEX. They also tested the sensitivity and specificity of CAMCOG compared to the MMSE for detecting organic mental impairment. They observed that the MMSE (cut-off value of 21/22) had a sensitivity of 96% and a specificity of 80% whereas CAMCOG (cut-off value of 79/80) yielded a sensitivity of 92% and a specificity of 96%. Thus the MMSE is slightly more sensitive but less specific than CAMCOG.

One of the major advantages of CAMDEX is that it provides adequate information to achieve a variety of diagnoses according to operational diagnostic criteria (e.g. DSMIII). The diagnostic categories include four categories of dementia (senile dementia of the Alzheimer's type (SDAT), multi-infarct dementia, mixed SDAT and dementia secondary to other causes), two categories of clouding of consciousness or delirium, depression, anxiety or phobic disorder, and paranoid or paraphrenic illness (the latter are psychotic disorders developing for the first time in older life).

Screening for cognitive decline in the elderly

The Mini Mental State Examination (MMSE) (Folstein *et al.* 1975) is the most commonly used screen for cognitive decline in dementia and is used both clinically and for research. The MMSE is divided into two sections and takes about 10 minutes to complete. The first section requires vocal responses only and covers orientation, memory and attention, and can result in a maximum score of 21. The second section tests the ability to name,

Table 8.6. Interviews and questionnaires used with elderly subjects.

Name	Author(s)	Type of interview/ questionnaire	Subject (S) or informant (I)	Symptoms or problems covered
CAMDEX	Roth et al. 1986	Comprehensive interview + cognitive test	S and I	Diagnoses in DSMIV activity cognition
CAMCOG	Roth et al. 1986	Screener	S	Cognition
MMSE	Folstein et al. 1975	Screener	S	Cognition
Blessed DRS	Blessed et al. 1968	Screener	S	Cognition
Mattis DRS	Sahy et al. 1991	Screener	S	Cognition
BEHAVE-AD	Reisburg et al. 1987	Interview	I	Psychopathology activity, behaviour
NPI	Cummins et al. 1994	Interview	I	Psychopathology behaviour
MOUSEPAD	Allen and Burns 1996	Semi-structured interview	I	Psychopathology (ex depression) behaviour
PBE	Hope and Fairburn 1992	Detailed and lengthy interview	I	Behaviour
Cornell scale	Alexopoulos et al. 1988	Interviews	S and I	Depression in dementia

Table 8.6. (Continued)

Name	Author(s)	Type of interview/ questionnaire	Subject (S) or informant (I)	Symptoms or problems covered
Geriatric Mental Status Schedule	Copeland et al. 1987	Interview (community use)	S	Depression anxiety and other disorders in community settings
Bristol ADLS	Bucks et al. 1996	Informant report scale	I	Daily living activities
Cleveland SADL	Patterson et al. 1992	Informant report scale (community use)	I	Daily living activities
FAST	Scian and Reisburg 1992	Informant report scale	I	Daily living activities
CDR	Morris 1993	Comprehensive structured interview	S and I	Global severity of Alzheimer's
GDS	Reisburg et al. 1982	Severity scale	I (expert)	Global severity of Alzheimer's
TSI	Albert and Cohen 1992	Observational test	I	Severity of severe Alzheimer's
M-OSPD	Auer et al. 1994	Observational test	I	Severity of severe Alzheimer's
SIB	Saxton et al. 1990	Observational test	I	Severity of severe Alzheimer's

(Cont.)

Table 8.6. (*Continued*)

Name	Author(s)	Type of interview/ questionnaire	Subject (S) or informant (I)	Symptoms or problems covered
HIS	Hachinski *et al.* 1975	Observational test	I	Differentiating vascular from Alzheimer's
FTD	Lebert *et al.* 1998	Observational test	I	Differentiating frontotemporal from Alzheimer's

CAMDEX   Cambridge Mental Disorders of the Elderly Examination
CAMCOG   Cambridge Cognitive Examination
MMSE   Mini Mental State Examination
Blessed DRS   Blessed Dementia Rating Scale
Mattis DRS   Mattis Dementia Rating Scale
BEHAVE-AD   Behavioural Pathology in Alzheimer's Disease Rating Scale
NPI   Neuropsychiatric Inventory
MOUSEPAD   Manchester + Oxford University Scale for the Psychopathological Assessment of Dementia
PBE   Present Behavioural Examination
Bristol ADLS   Bristol Activities of Daily Living Scale
Cleveland SADL   Cleveland Scale of Activities of Daily Living
FAST   Functional Assessment Staging Test
CDR   Clinical Dementia Rating Scale
GDS   Global Deterioration Scale
TSI   Test for Severe Impairment
M-OSPD   Modified Ordinal Scales of Psychological Development
SIB   Severe Impairment Battery
HIS   Hachinski Ischaemic Score
FTD   Fronto-temporal Behavioural Scale

follow verbal unwritten commands, write a sentence spontaneously, and copy a complex polygon, and can produce a maximum score of 9. The combined maximum total score is therefore 30. The MMSE is not intended to replace a complete clinical appraisal in reaching a final diagnosis of dementia, for example, and can be used to assess cognition in a variety of populations, although it is mainly applied to the elderly. The MMSE has good test/retest reliability (Folstein *et al.* 1975), but it does show small learning effects when tests are administered close together (i.e. two weeks apart) (Doraiswamy and Kaiser 2000). It has been validated against a number of criteria, for example, concurrent validity was shown between the MMSE and the Wechsler Adult Intelligence Scale, verbal and performance scores, producing significant correlations of with verbal and performance IQ (Folstein *et al.* 1975). However, the relationship with IQ can cause changes in sensitivity for those with high or low premorbid IQs and modifications to the MMSE have been suggested to improve sensitivity in these groups (Murden and Galbraith 1997; Leopold and Borson 1997). The MMSE is highly sensitive to the detection of dementia in the elderly (Roth *et al.* 1986, Rait *et al.* 2000), but has less specificity when compared to a number of non-dementing elderly diagnostic groups (Roth *et al.* 1986; Rait *et al.* 2000). To improve specificity for Alzheimer's disease, Yuspeh and colleagues (Yuspeh *et al.* 1998) modified the three-item recall portion of the MMSE, by replacing it with a queued recall procedure which increased specificity for the detection of Alzheimer's disease in relation to subcortical vascular ischemic dementia and unaffected controls. The MMSE has been used widely and is translated into a number of languages (Cappeliez *et al.* 1996; Tosnerova and Bahbouh 1998). The MMSE has also been adapted for use as a telephone interview (Monterio *et al.* 1998). Although the MMSE is the most popular screen for cognition in the elderly other measures are in use, which include the Blessed Dementia Rating Scale (Blessed *et al.* 1968), the Mattis Dementia Rating Scale (Shay *et al.* 1991), and the CAMCOG. In addition, a clock-drawing test has also been used as a quick screen of cognitive abilities.

Measuring behavioural disturbance, depression, and activities of daily living in the elderly

It has become increasingly apparent that cognitive decline is not the only feature associated with dementia in the elderly. Psychopathology, such as hallucinations and delusions (Burns *et al.* 1990), and disturbances of behaviour, such as wandering (Allen and Burns 1995) are also common. There are a number of measures that specifically assess these aspects of psychopathology in the elderly. We will consider three here: the Behavioural Pathology in Alzheimer's Disease Rating Scale (BEHAVE-AD) (Reisberg *et al.* 1987), the Neuro Psychiatric Inventory (NPI) (Cummins *et al.* 1994) and the Manchester and Oxford University Scale for the Psychopathological Assessment of Dementia (MOUSEPAD) (Allen and Burns 1995). Because of the cognitive problems in patients, all the scales reviewed here rely on information from carers.

The BEHAVE-AD is divided into two sections, the first assesses symptomatology which includes delusions, hallucinations, activity disturbances, anxieties and phobias, and the second attempts a global rating of these areas, indicating severity (Reisberg *et al.* 1987). The BEHAVE-AD has been criticized for using aggressive behaviour as a severity indicator for rating delusions and misidentifications as well as rating it separately, which can lead to duplication in recording. It also includes phenomenology related to physical illness, such as delirium.

The Neuro Psychiatric Inventory (NPI) covers twelve neuropsychiatric domains: delusions, hallucinations, agitation/aggression, dysphoria/depression, anxiety, euphoria/elation, apathy/indifference, disinhibition, irritability, aberrant motor behaviour, night-time behavioural disturbances and eating disturbances (Cummins *et al.* 1994. Each domain is sampled by an initial screening question, followed by specific questions if the screening is answered positively. Items are rated in terms of both their frequency (1–4) and severity (1–3), which together yield a composite symptom domain score. The NPI is delivered in the form of an interview with a carer. However, a questionnaire based on the NPI has also been developed (NPI-Q, Kaufer *et al.* 2000), which is quick to administer and correlates well with the NPI. However, the NPI-Q is slightly more sensitive to detecting hallucinations, whereas the NPI is more sensitive to delusions. Both scales show a good test re-test reliability and convergent validity with respect to individual and total domain scores.

The MOUSEPAD is a semi-structured interview for use by interviewers with psychiatric or psychological experience and is the only one of the measures described here which has a glossary (Allen and Burns 1995). The domains covered include delusions, hallucinations, misidentifications, and behavioural changes including walking, eating, sleeping, aggression, laughing/crying. The measure does not cover depression. The frequency and severity of the behaviours or symptoms are assessed using two time frames; the last month and over the course of the dementia syndrome. Inter-rater reliability is generally good, although the measure only shows adequate to low test re-test reliability (Allen and Burns, 1995). Allen and Burns also report kappas of between 0.43 and 0.67 for a test of concurrent validity using the Present Behavioural Examination (PBE) (Hope and Fairburn, 1992). The PBE has a similar structure to MOUSEPAD, but provides a far more detailed account of behaviour and accordingly is probably too long for most research and clinical settings.

Depression and dementia are the two most common psychiatric syndromes observed in the elderly and since depression can result in transitory cognitive problems, it can be misdiagnosed as dementia. Although some measures include depression (e.g. NPI and CAMDEX) the Cornell Scale is one of the few to test specifically for depression in dementia (Alexopoulos *et al.* 1988). The Scale has nineteen items and covers mood related signs, behavioural disturbance, physical signs, and ideational disturbances associated with depression. It is intended that a clinician or researcher with psychiatric knowledge administer the interview, and information is obtained from both the subject and a knowledgeable observer (usually a member of the nursing staff). Items are rated in terms of severity (0-2). The Cornell Scale has good inter-rater reliability, internal consistency and sensitivity (Alexopoulos *et al.* 1988) as well as good concurrent validity when compared with Research Diagnostic Criteria.

A structured interview and computerized scoring system specifically devised for epidemiological studies of mental disorder in the elderly is the Geriatric Mental Status Schedule (GMS) and the computer-derived diagnostic system (AGECAT) (Copeland *et al.* 1987). This system has been used in a large epidemiological study of the over 65-year-olds living in Liverpool. The DIS (see chapter 5) and CES-D (see chapter 7) have also been used to evaluate the rates of mental disorder in the elderly living in the community (Johnson *et al.* 1992).

To achieve a diagnosis of dementia it is important to establish that cognitive decline significantly interferes with the person's work, usual social activity or relationships with others. Accordingly, a number of scales have been developed to measure these activities. A good example is the Bristol Activities of Daily Living Scale produced by Bucks and colleagues (Bucks *et al.* 1996, Byrne *et al.* 2000). This scale is brief and easy to administer and can be completed by carers. It measures activities associated with eating, drinking, dressing, personal hygiene, orientation in time and space, communication, housework, shopping, finances, hobbies and transport.

Patients are rated in relation to premorbid functioning on a scale that assesses severity (0–3). The scale shows good test re-test reliability, concurrent validity with the MMSE and good sensitivity to changes over time (Bucks *et al.* 1996; Byrne *et al.* 2000).

Of the numerous scales developed to assess activities of daily living (Ramsey *et al.* 1995) only two measure functional ability and were designed for community use. These are the Cleveland Scale of Activities of Daily Living (CSADL) (Patterson *et al.* 1992) and the Functional Assessment Staging Test (FAST) (Scian and Reisburg 1992).

Measures of specific forms of dementia

Global Measures of Severity in Alzheimer's Disease

A number of scales have been developed to rate global severity of Alzheimer's disease. These include the Clinical Dementia Rating Scale (CDR) (Morris 1993) and the Global Deterioration Scale (GDS) (Reisburg *et al.* 1982). The CDR is based on a comprehensive structured interview with the patient and an informant. Performance is rated in six domains: memory, orientation, judgement and problem solving, community activities, home and hobbies and personal care. The GDS is a 7-point scale of severity describing stages of dementia from normal (1) to late dementia (7). It is assessed by an individual with psychiatric knowledge who can work from a variety of information sources. However, it is becoming apparent that many of the observational tests of the later stages of Alzheimer's disease suffer a ceiling effect when assessing cognitive variables. A series of other tests have been proposed to address this and include the Test for Severe Impairment (TSI) (Albert and Cohen, 1992), the modified Ordinal Scales of Psychological Development (M-OSPD) (Auer *et al.* 1994) and the Severe Impairment Battery (SIB) (Saxton *et al.* 1990). All these tests show good test re-test reliability and the SIB has also been shown to be sensitive to change measured longitudinally (Panisset *et al.* 1994).

Measuring vascular dementia

The Hachinski Ischemic Score (HIS) is probably the most widely used scale to differentiate patients with vascular dementia from those with more common dementias such as Alzheimer's disease (Hachinski *et al.* 1975). The HIS was devised by relating various symptoms and signs of dementia to

Table 8.7. Hachinski Ischaemic Scores (HIS) for differentiating vascular (multi-infarct) from Alzheimer's type dementia.

Clinical feature	Weighted score
Abrupt onset	2
Stepwise deterioration	1
Fluctuating course	2
Nocturnal confusion	1
Preserved personality	1
Depression	1
Somatic complaints	1
Emotional incontinence	1
Hypertension	1
History of strokes	2
Associated arteriosclerosis	1
Focal neurological signs	2
Focal neurological symptoms	2

measures of cerebral blood flow. The subjects with dementia were divided into two groups; those with high and low cerebral blood flow. It was assumed that high cerebral blood flow was associated with vascular disease, while those with low flow had Alzheimer's type dementia. Each clinical feature was given a weighted score, which are summated to give the HIS. A score of less than 4 indicates an Alzheimer's type picture while a score above 7, a vascular or multi-infarct dementia.

Since it was first published, the HIS has been revised and refined (Small 1985). In a recent meta-analysis, Moroney and colleagues (Moroney *et al.* 1997) showed that the HIS differed significantly amongst groups with pathologically verified Alzheimer's disease, multi-infarct dementia and mixed dementia. Receiver operated characteristic curves (see chapter 4) confirmed the original cut-off points of ≤ 4 for Alzheimer's dementia and ≥ 7 for multi-infarct dementia, with sensitivity of 89% and specificity of 89.3%. Sensitivity was similar in comparisons with mixed dementia but specificity was reduced for both multi-infarct and Alzheimer's disease.

Measuring frontotemporal dementia

The Frontotemporal Behavioural Scale is a recent example of a scale developed to differentiate frontotemporal dementia (FTD) from Alzheimer's disease and vascular dementia. The score on the scale was found to be higher in FTD than in other dementias. With a cut-off of 3 points on the scale, FTD patients were diagnosed with a specificity of 95% and sensitivity of 91% (Lebert *et al.* 1998).

The classification of psychopathology associated with substance misuse and the diagnostic interviews and rating scales used for evaluation

The rising rate of abuse and dependence of street drugs and alcohol in many Western countries, has become a major public health issue. Such misuse is frequently associated with physical and mental health problems, as well as much personal suffering both to the individual and their families. Many psychopathological symptoms can be caused by substance misuse. For example, ecstasy, an amphetamine-like substance, can cause hallucinations and delusions similar to those found in schizophrenia or mania. Schizophrenia-like psychotic illnesses may also be associated with heavy use of cannabis. Depression and anxiety are often associated with drug and alcohol withdrawal, and death by suicide or accident is more frequent than in non-abusing members of the general population.

As well as these psychological symptoms, misuse of drugs or alcohol is also associated with impaired functioning (e.g. at work or in caring for a young family), criminal behaviour, and physical harm. Those who inject drugs such as heroin or cocaine are also at additional increased risk of catching the Human Immunodeficiency Virus (HIV) through the sharing of contaminated needles.

The operational definitions for substance misuse in ICD10 and DSMIV reflect these additional areas of symptomatology. Table 8.8 shows the ICD10 classification of 'Mental and Behavioural Disorders due to Psychoactive Substance Use' (F10–F19) (WHO 1993).

The same categories are also in DSMIV, although here the order is alphabetical (alcohol, amphetamine caffeine etc. through to sedatives/hypnotics). In addition, DSMIV has separate categories for 'use disorder' i.e. dependence and abuse, and 'drug-induced disorder' e.g. depression, or anxiety due to drug use. For example, 304.40 is assigned to 'amphetamine dependence', while 292.0 relates to amphetamine intoxication and 292.89 to 'amphetamine-induced anxiety disorder'.

Although these operational definitions of psychoactive substance misuse have undoubtedly improved diagnostic reliability, and ensured that

Table 8.8. ICD10: Mental and behavioural disorders due to psychoactive substance use.

F10: alcohol	F13: sedatives/ hypnotics	F16: hallucinogens
F11: opioids	F14: cocaine	F17: tobacco (nicotine)
F12: cannabis	F15: other stimulants (caffeine)	F18: volatile substances (inhalants)
		F19: multiple (polysubstance) use

Fourth and fifth character, (e.g. F10.XX), specify the clinical condition, i.e. acute intoxication, harmful use, dependence.

epidemiological surveys are reasonably comparable cross-nationally, there remain problems related to the definitions of terms such as 'problem use', 'addiction', 'dependence' and 'craving' (Nutt and Law 2000). In the case of craving, a questionnaire method has been devised in an attempt to tease apart the various components of the symptom, in order to improve diagnostic precision (Tiffany *et al.* 1993).

The evaluation of the psychopathology associated with substance misuse has taken on national importance in a number of countries. The interviews devised to evaluate the broad range of psychopathology also include sections for the assessment of drugs and alcohol (e.g. SCAN, CIDI, SADS, SCID, and DIGS – see chapter 5). However, detailed diagnostic interviews, specific to the study of those with psychopathology associated with substance misuse, have also been devised. Probably the most well known and in current use are the Semi-Structured Assessment for the Genetics of Alcohol (SSAGA), and the Composite International Diagnostic Interview, Substance Abuse Module (CIDI-SAM)(Cottler *et al.* 1989, Cottler *et al.* 1991) (for further details about web site address for SSAGA see appendix).

Screening for alcohol misuse

It is also important to screen for alcohol misuse and dependence in various settings, in particular primary care and general hospitals. In such settings, an individual's physical health problems may be due to, or complicated by, excess consumption of or withdrawal from alcohol. For example, excess alcohol consumption can cause high blood pressure, raised levels of liver enzymes or enlarged red blood cells. Also, confusional states or *delirium* can be caused by alcohol withdrawal (e.g. when someone is admitted to a general medical ward, and cannot obtain their usual 'dose' of alcohol). The physical concomitants of excess alcohol consumption can be used to validate various rating scales for alcohol misuse. For example, conventional blood tests including mean corpuscular volume and liver function tests, such as the gamma-glutamyl transferase level have been used to validate self report screening questionnaires (Leouffe *et al.* 1990, Aertgeerts *et al.* 2001, Schneekloth *et al.* 2001).

Such screening questionnaires include the Michigan Alcoholism Screening Test (MAST) (Powers and Spickard 1984, Leouffe *et al.* 1990), a 24-item yes/no self report questionnaire used in hospital outpatients, the Alcohol Use Disorders Identification Test (AUDIT) (Saunders *et al.* 1993), a 10-item brief structured self-report questionnaire for use in primary care settings, the Self-Administered Alcoholism Screening Test (SAAST) (Pristach *et al.* 1993) also used with hospitalized subjects, and the four-item CAGE questionnaire (Ewing 1984). The latter is especially useful to the busy clinician, since there are just four easily remembered questions. Any positive response raises the suspicion of high alcohol consumption and or problems associated with consumption. The questions relate to: (i) 'cutting down' (C), 'have you ever wanted to cut down on your consumption of alcohol but been unable to?', (ii) 'annoyed' (A), 'have you ever been annoyed by criticism of your drinking?', (iii) 'guilty' (G), 'have you ever felt guilty about your alcohol consumption?', and (iv) 'eye opener' (E), 'have you ever needed a drink to get you going first thing in the morning?'. More recently another short screening questionnaire has been produced consisting of an amalgamation of two questions from AUDIT and three from CAGE. The 'Five Shot' questionnaire, (Seppa *et al.* 1998) has been shown to be efficient in differentiating between moderate and heavy drinkers. The Five Shot and AUDIT were shown to perform well in screening primary care attenders for early alcohol abuse or dependence when compared against blood tests confirming excess alcohol use (Aertgeerts *et al.* 2001).

There are also several questionnaires that evaluate the consequences of alcohol use such as the Alcohol Problems Questionnaire (Drummond 1990). The Addiction Severity Index (ASI) (McLellan *et al.* 1980) can be used to assess both the consequences of use as well as evaluate severity of dependence. Other scales that measure the severity of alcohol dependence include the Severity of Alcohol Dependence Scale (SADS) (Stockwell *et al.* 1979), and the Short Alcohol Dependence Data (SADD) (Davidson *et al.* 1989).

Evaluation of the psychopathology associated with eating disorders

Predominately affecting young women, anorexia nervosa and the bingeing disorders bulimia and bulimia nervosa have become increasingly prevalent in Western countries since the 1950s (Russell 2000). The key clinical feature of both types of disorder is an overwhelming desire to weigh less. In anorexia, this is achieved by stringent dieting that leads to excessive and unhealthy weight loss. In the bulimic disorders, the ability to abstain from food consumption, although desired, is not achieved. Indeed there may be bouts of excessive eating (bingeing) which then leads to self-induced vomiting or purgation (use of laxatives) to get rid of the effects of the food consumed. Consequently, the effects of starvation influence the psychopathology associated with anorexia, while the bingeing/purging/vomiting cycles that typify bulimia lead to metabolic abnormalities (for example, low blood potassium levels) that complicate the psychopathological profile.

Both anorexia and bulimia are frequently associated with depression and anxiety, as well as alcohol abuse (more especially bulimia). As in the case of substance misuse disorders, eating disorders psychopathology is included in the general psychiatric interviews we have already reviewed, such as SCAN and CIDI. In addition, the Eating Disorders Examination (Fairburn and Cooper 1993) provides a more specific clinical evaluation. Two self-report questionnaires have also been widely used as screeners; the Eating Attitudes Test (EAT) (Garner and Garfinkel 1979) and the Eating Disorders Inventory (Garner 1991).

Evaluation of the psychopathology associated with childbirth

While pregnancy is for most women a time relatively free from mental disorder, an excess of psychopathology is associated with the postnatal period (i.e. up to one year following the birth of a child). The 'baby blues' is a transient period of tearfulness and low mood that occurs between 3 and 10 days postpartum, and although present in about one third of all new mothers, the symptoms are brief and self-limiting in the majority. However, a proportion of mothers, goes on to develop a more severe postnatal depression, while between one in 500 to one in a thousand will develop a psychotic illness termed 'puerperal psychosis'. It is vitally important for the health of both mother and child that these more severe forms of mental disorder are rapidly identified and treated. Consequently, a quick screening self-report questionnaire has been devised specifically to evaluate the severity of depressive symptoms occurring in the postnatal period. The Edinburgh Post Natal Depression Rating Scale (EPDS) (Cox *et al.* 1987) has been validated against Research Diagnostic Criteria for depression applied via a clinical interview. The authors considered that the screener could be used in the secondary prevention of postnatal depression. While some authors have shown that the EPDS is superior in eliciting depression in postnatal subjects, when compared with the Beck Depression Inventory (Harris *et al.* 1989), others have found poor agreement between four different self-report questionnaires used in such individuals (Condon and Corkindale 1997). The authors suggest that their findings reflect the differences in the item content of the questionnaires, which in turn reflects the notions of depression held by the designers of the questionnaires. Not with standing such criticisms, the EPDS has enjoyed wide international use in postnatal populations and has been translated into a number of languages.

In this chapter we have reviewed the psychopathology found in children, adolescents, the elderly cognitively impaired, those with low intellectual abilities, those misusing psychoactive substances, and individuals who have an eating disorder or who develop a mental disorder after giving birth. Of necessity, we have been brief and rather selective about what we have included. Consequently we recommend readers to the references cited, and other texts if more detailed information is required.

In chapter 9 we will review the measurement of personality, both normal and pathological (personality disorder), and how this relates to and influences the presentation of mental disorders.

Personality and Personality Disorders

Introduction

In this chapter, we tackle personality and personality disorders, a subject seen by some as the most difficult and contentious area of measurement in psychopathology. The term 'personality' refers to the behavioural attributes that characterize individuals and differentiate them from others. Terms to describe personality, such as 'extravert' (being outgoing and gregarious) or 'neurotic' (being anxious and worried), have entered everyday language. The notion that personality can cause problems for the individual or others, or deviate from what is considered normal, underpins the concept of a 'personality disorder'. For example, an extremely perfectionistic individual may be so preoccupied with the details, rules, lists, order and organization of their daily life that they become unable to complete any tasks or do their job effectively. The *anankastic* or *obsessional* features of their personality are so extreme as to cause impairment of function, and the subject is then diagnosed as having 'anankastic personality disorder' (WHO 1993).

Historically, the difficulties in measuring personality disorders have been exacerbated and complicated by the separation between those researchers, mainly academic psychologists, who have attempted to conceptualize and devise measures of 'normal' personality *traits*, and those mainly from a clinical background, who have sought to describe and classify personality *disorders*. It is only comparatively recently that there has been recognition that this division is not helpful. Here we will try to briefly describe and integrate these two strands, before describing the measures that are currently available to classify and assess personality disorders.

What is Personality?

Personality can be defined as the individual's entire repertoire of relatively stable and enduring behaviours. Conventionally cognitive characteristics, that is intellect and memory, are considered separately so that personality and cognition are the 'big two' domains in the study of individual differences. As with all classification schema, this has a degree of arbitrariness. However, at the level of behavioural description, the constituents of personality and cognition overlap little, so that the division between personality and cognitive domains remains a useful one.

Implicit in the concept of personality as stable and enduring is the idea that an assessment of personality provides a basis for prediction of behaviour in the future. Hence disorders of personality are usually seen as reflecting enduring traits rather than transient or alterable states that may change over time. This distinction is recognized in the multiaxial organization of DSMIV, (see chapter 3) whereby Axis I consists of clinical disorders (and 'other conditions that may be a focus of clinical attention') and disorders of personality are included in a separate axis, Axis II. (This axis also includes mental retardation).

In both DSMIV and ICD10 personality disorders are classified according to distinct categories, and this has a straightforward and intuitive appeal. It fits with traditional clinical approaches where disorders generally are seen as more or less discrete entities, as well as with an everyday common sense view of personality that tends to categorize people into *types*. However, as we shall see, the results of applying typologies to personality within the normal range are less satisfactory than allowing that individuals show variation along continuous dimensions or *traits*.

Historical attempts to describe personality types

There is a tendency in everyday life to pick out some relevant characteristics that we think describe an individual and use these to sum up their personality in a global fashion. This has probably ever been the case. From the time of Hippocrates in the fifth century BC until the seventeenth century, (Burton 1652) personality was considered as being caused by a blending of the four bodily *humours,* and individuals were described according to which of four humours predominated. *Melancholic* individuals in whom black bile predominated showed a tendency to worry and depression; whereas *choleric* individuals were irritable and active; a result of yellow bile predominating. *Phlegmatic* individuals, thought to have an excess of phlegm, were unmoved by emotion, whereas in *sanguine* individuals, where blood was the principle humour, the main characteristics were hopefulness and optimism. Needless to say, although this classification scheme interested early experimental psychologists such as Wundt (1903), it was not one that lent itself to empirical verification.

Nevertheless, attempts to categorize personality according to other physical characteristics, such as the size and locations of bony protuberances on the head (*phrenology*) and more recently the size and shape of the body, have continued into the twentieth century (Porter 1997). The *body type* classification of personality was introduced by Kretschmer (1936) and later modified by Sheldon *et al.* (1942). This theory proposed that there were three main body types; *endomorphs, mesomorphs* and *ectomorphs,* related to which of the three primitive embryonic layers predominated. Endomorphs were round with well-developed features, and were said to show sociability, affection and a love of comfort. Mesomorphs had an athletic build and were characterized by energetic, domineering personalities. Ectomorphs were slim and fine featured and had a predominantly 'cerebrotonic' personality, that is, one characterized by restraint, sensitivity and shyness. Although Sheldon based this typology on an attempt to classify body types using photographs of student volunteers, and claimed a strong correlation between body types and the supposed personality characteristics, the objectivity of those methods was called into question, and his approaches did not stand the test of time.

A somewhat more enduring twentieth century typology was based upon Freudian theory (Freud 1904). This proposed that personalities could be classified according to the phase of development in which an individual was 'fixated'. Those who were fixated at the *oral* stage are either 'oral sadistic' with a gloomy and malicious outlook or 'oral passive', those who are dependent but tend to become hostile if their needs are not gratified. Those who are fixated at the *anal* stage of development show obsessional characteristics, such as stubbornness, parsimony and orderliness. According to Freud, such characteristics were acquired as a result of toilet training, and an accentuated interest in control over the bowels.

Those fixated at the *phallic* stage are self interested, narcissistic showoffs and, like those showing predominantly oral or anal characteristics, have failed to progress to the mature *genital* level of adjustment. Although such categorization may be at a metaphorical level, they are clearly not easy to subject to scientific scrutiny, and even the most devoted Freudians conceded that in practice most individuals have the capacity at various times to show mixtures of 'oral', 'anal' or 'phallic' tendencies.

Types versus traits (categories versus dimensions)

A post-Freudian typology that has been more influential and enduring in influencing personality theory was proposed by Jung (1923). This described individuals as being either *introvert* – those for whom their inner mental life is more salient that their external environment – or *extravert* – those who show a predominantly outwardly directed consciousness. A somewhat modified version of these Jungian concepts was adopted by Eysenck and Eysenck (1963) and subsequently by other personality theorists as a basis for an extraversion-introversion dimension. To some extent, Jung and the other influential typologists such as Kretschmer and Sheldon recognized that the personality types that they described actually had dimensional components. Indeed, the second half of the twentieth century saw a major shift away from typologies towards the development of structural models of personality based upon dimensional traits.

Pioneers of this approach were Hans and Sybil Eysenck (Eysenck and Eysenck 1975), who proposed that personality could be measured along three dimensions – extraversion–introversion, neuroticism–stability and psychoticism, and Cattell, who proposed a more complicated system in which personality varies along sixteen different dimensions (Cattell 1973). Both Eysenck and Eysenck (1975) and Cattell (1973) derived their dimensional traits using a *factor analytical* statistical approach. Briefly, this method starts out with a large number of items describing personality, usually responses to self-report questionnaires, and examines the correlations between these items. Subsequently factors are extracted from the correlation matrix in the form of dimensions that maximize the similarity between items loading on one particular factor while, at the same time, maximizing the differences between factors. More recently, there has been considerable debate as to how many factors are needed to adequately describe personality, and there is now a general consensus in support of five dimensions.

The Big Five

The main personality factors are often called the 'Big Five', on account of the breadth of features encompassed within each dimension. They are; *openness to experience, conscientiousness, extraversion, agreeableness* and *neuroticism* (Costa and McCrae 1992). These personality dimensions, for which the word OCEAN provides useful nemonic, are summarized and further described in table 9.1.

Table 9.1. The 'Big Five' dimension of personality.

Trait	Description of high scorers	Description of low scorers
Openness to experience	Diverse interests, curious, enjoys novel ideas	Rigid, dislikes change, conventional
Conscientiousness	Organized, dependable, thorough	Careless, poor planning skills
Extraversion	Active, outgoing, socially at ease, many friends	Shy, anxious in new company
Agreeableness	Trusting, modest, compliant, helpful, easily taken advantage of	Stubborn, argumentative, unforgiving
Neuroticism	Anxious, worrying, pessimistic, lacking self confidence	Relaxed, stable, copes well with adversity

Although there is now reasonable international agreement that there are five main personality dimensions in adults, two additional dimensions have been described in children and adolescents (John *et al.* 1994). The additional dimensions proposed as occurring in children are *irritability* and *activity* (John *et al.* 1994, Luby *et al.* 1999, Moore and Farmer 2002).

Personality as a result of 'person–situation interactions'

Although describing personality in terms of dimensional traits is widely accepted, critics of trait theory have pointed out that individuals do not behave in a social vacuum: rather they respond to situations and their behaviours may differ from one situation to another. For example, someone who appears outgoing and extravert in one set of circumstances may appear more socially inhibited in another. Thus, personality might be better seen as resulting from a complex series of 'person–situation interactions'. However, scores on measures of personality traits represent average effects, so that someone's score on a scale such as extraversion reflects a typical response over a range of situations. In fact, the current five-factor theory of personality (McCrae and Costa 1999) allows that 'social and physical environment interacts with personality dispositions to shape characteristic adaptations'. Furthermore, the theory allows that individuals both selectively influence the environment and that a perception of the environment and the way it is construed is also influenced by personality. This is in keeping with modern behavioural genetic approaches to personality that no longer assume that the individual is the passive reception of environmental influences but instead propose that personality results from a complex gene-environment interplay (Plomin and Caspi 1995).

Temperament and character: A bio-psychosocial approach to personality

Also, in response to the idea that environmental influences, such as developmental factors, life experiences and learning have an impact on the basic genetically influenced traits of personality, Cloninger (1987) proposed a unified bio-psychosocial theory of temperament and personality development. In this theory, personality is conceptualized 'as a combination of heritable, neuro-biologically based traits (temperament dimensions), and traits reflecting socio-cultural learning (character dimensions)'. The *temperament dimensions* are thought to be related to activity in specific central neurotransmitter systems (Peirson *et al.* 1999) and have been termed, *harm avoidance, novelty seeking, reward dependence,* and *persistence*. Harm avoidance refers to 'a tendency to respond intensely to signals of aversive stimuli' leading to cautious, inhibited and apprehensive behaviour in high scoring individuals. Thus there is some commonality with neuroticism. In contrast, novelty-seeking is conceptualized as 'a heritable tendency toward intense exhilaration or excitement in response to novel stimuli', and has an overlap with extraversion.

The *character dimensions* described by Cloninger (1987) are *self-directedness, cooperativeness* and *self-transcendence*. Cloninger and colleagues (1993) also proposed that these seven temperament and character dimensions could be related to psychopathology. A version of the TCI for children has also been produced (Luby *et al.* 1999).

Types of tests and issues of reliability and validity

The concepts of reliability and validity are discussed in greater detail in chapter 4, but here we are concerned with the specifics of tests of personality. Some early attempts to measure personality took the form of *projective tests*. The two best known are the *Rorschach* test (Oberholzer 1924) and the *Thematic Apperception Test* (TAT) (Murray 1943). The Rorschach method was to present subjects with a series of inkblocks and asked them to describe what they see in each of them. The basic assumption is that, presented with these ambiguous stimuli, subjects will describe them in a way that reflects their underlying personality structure. In the TAT, subjects were given series of black and white pictures showing a variety of scenes and were then asked what is happening in the picture, what events might have led up to the scene that is depicted and what the subject think is likely to happen next. Both tests relied originally on psychoanalytic concepts and suffered greatly from lack of reproducibility or reliability. That is, there was inevitably a great deal of subjectivity on the part of the person administering the test as to what an individual's responses meant.

Modern personality tests usually take the form of a self-report procedure, most often a questionnaire or 'paper and pencil' test. Although this sounds more prosaic than the older projective tests, questionnaires have a virtue of allowing reliability to be evaluated, and of having their validity open to scrutiny.

Questionnaires usually rely on a forced choice where the subject responds yes or no to each item. Initially, questions are usually chosen because of their *content validity,* that is, that the item appears to represent a measure of some aspect of personality (see chapter 4). However, there are problems of interpretation if subjects' responses are taken at face value. For example, it is important that items are not constructed in an ambiguous way that will tend to give misleading or unreliable results. There is also a problem that some subjects may, deliberately or unconsciously, falsify their response. The most common tendency is to respond to questions in a way that seems *socially desirable.* To take this into account, some tests such as the Eysenck Personality Questionnaire (EPQ) (Eysenck and Eysenck 1975) incorporate a *social desirability* or *lie* scale. For example, positively endorsing an item such as 'I would never tell a lie under any circumstances whatsoever' is almost certainly a lie! However, some respondents may perceive this, as the 'socially correct' response and mark it as 'true'.

Tending to conform to social desirability can be described as a type of *response set.* Other recognized response sets in questionnaires are 'yes saying' or acquiescence and 'no saying' or deviance. Acquiescence is the tendency to select a 'yes' response to a disproportionate number of items in a questionnaire (and may in itself sometimes be associated to particular personality type, a form of agreeableness). Deviance, on the other hand, is a tendency to respond to items in an unusual or non-conforming way. A more mundane form of *response set* may occur when all of the items in the questionnaire measuring a particular trait require the same reply. For example, if all of the items on a questionnaire to do with worrying or anxiety require the reply 'yes', some individuals at the outset of answering such a questionnaire may decide, having responded 'no' to the first few items, to continue to respond in the same way throughout the rest of the questionnaire. In order to avoid *response set,* it is therefore usual to mix items such that a proportion aiming to measure a particular trait require a proportion of positive and negative responses. For example, a 'positive' item measuring neuroticism might be 'I always tend to worry a lot' and a negative one 'I am not easily upset'.

In addition to overcoming the problems of *response set,* properties of a useful personality test should include high internal consistency, which in effect is the same as internal reliability as measured for example by Cronbach's alpha, and good stability as reflected in test re-test agreement (see chapter 4). In practice, the stability of personality measures such as the Big Five tends to be good in healthy subjects, but the main confounding factor in clinical populations is *mood state*. For example, most individuals tend to be less extraverted and more neurotic when they are in a depressed state than when they are recovered.

In addition to face validity and content validity, it is desirable that a personality measure or scale has *construct* validity. Construct validity depends upon there being some underlying explanatory theory in which the trait to be measured is an intervening variable or construct. Such an explanatory theory should help in making prediction about future behaviour. For example, predictions may be made about the physiological or behavioural correlates about a measure or about the extent that scores on a particular measure reflect susceptibility to psychological disorder or distress. A somewhat different approach is to use *criterion keying*, where tests are constructed on the basis of their ability to distinguish between certain apparently well-defined groups. For example, the Minnesota Multiphasic Personality Inventory (MMPI) (Hathaway and McKinley 1951) is a classic example where criterion keying has been used to construct scales that relate to the symptoms of various psychiatric disorders.

Questionnaire measures of personality dimensions

Table 9.2 summarizes the main features of five different dimensional personality measures. The Eysenck personality questionnaire (EPQ) (Eysenck and Eysenck 1975) is one of the most widely used scales for deriving measures of extraversion (E) and neuroticism (N), which have been the two most intensively studied of the Big Five. As mentioned, the EPQ also incorporates a 'lie' or social desirability scale and a fourth scale (P), which the Eysencks have called *psychoticism*. In fact the P-scale contains a mixture of items, some of which are to do with ideas of persecution and self-reference, whereas others reflect tough mindedness or psychopathy. More recently an additional fifth scale relating to addictive behaviour was added to the EPQ.

The NEO five factor inventory (NEO-FFI) (McCrae and Costa 1999) is a sixty-item questionnaire derived from an earlier, much longer set of scales that is specifically designed to measure the Big Five personality dimensions. It is probably the best known of current measures that cover all of the Big Five, but some other questionnaires currently in use include Goldberg's (1992) Trait Descriptive Adjectives (TDA) and the Big Five Inventory (BFI)

Table 9.2. Measures of personality.

Name	Author(s)	Traits measured	Format
Eysenck Personality Questionnaire (EPQ)	Eysenck and Eysenck 1975	Extraversion (E) Neuroticism (N) Psychoticism (P) Lie/social desirability (L)	90 yes/no items
NEO – Five Factor Inventory (NEO-FFI)	Costa and McCrae 1992	Big Five	60 items
Big Five Inventory (BFI)	John and Srivastava 1999	Big Five	44 questions with five-point Likert type response
Trait descriptive Adjectives (TDA)	Goldberg 1992	Big Five	100 adjectives, subjects endorse those that apply to them
Temperament and Character Inventory (TCI)	Cloninger *et al.* 1993	*Temperament:* harm avoidance, novelty seeking, reward dependence, persistence *Character:* self directedness, cooperativeness and self transcendence	226 yes/no items

(John *et al.* 1991). These three inventories show very good agreement in measuring extraversion, conscientiousness and neuroticism, but differ in terms of the resultant scores on agreeableness and openness (John and Srivastava 1999).

Cloninger's Temperament and Character Inventory (TCI) (Cloninger *et al.* 1993) is currently widely used, but differs conceptually from other questionnaires and in having a different terminology for its seven subscales (see above). Cloninger's measures are considerably influenced by clinical concepts, and he proposed that the TCI usually captures the dimensions that may be important in explaining psychopathology. A version of the TCI, the Junior Temperament and Character Inventory, has been devised for use with children (Luby *et al.* 1999).

As mentioned earlier, the MMPI is a set of scales that are even more explicitly designed to detect psychopathology, and is therefore regarded by some as a measure of personality disorder rather than personality within the normal range. Nevertheless, some of the MMPI subscales show a degree of overlap with the Big Five. For example, the *histrionic scale* relates to extraversion, the *paranoid scale* is to some extent the inverse of agreeableness, the *compulsive scale* is associated with conscientiousness, the *borderline scale* is associated with neuroticism and the *schizotypy scale* is the inverse of openness (John and Srivastava 1999).

Personality disorder

The current classification of personality disorders, in contrast with the prevailing view on how to measure and describe normal personality, relies entirely on categories or types rather than dimensions The definitions of personality disorder in DSMIV (American Psychiatric Association 1994) and ICD10 (World Health Organisation 1993) (see also chapter 3) are almost identical and define the term as denoting 'an enduring pattern of inner experience and behaviour that deviates markedly from the expectations of the individual's culture'. Both systems of classification recognise deviation in four particular areas.

1 *Cognition*, the way that the individual perceives and interprets the world and forms attitudes towards and images of their own self and others.

2 *Affectivity*, the range intensity and appropriateness of the individual's emotional responses.

3 *Interpersonal functioning*, the way that the individual relates to others and manages interactions with others.

4 *Impulse control*, the degree to which the individual can control impulses or delay gratification of needs.

Both DSM and ICD definitions require:

• That there are deviations in two or more of these areas,

• That the pattern is inflexible and pervasive across a broad range of situations; and

• That the pattern of behaviour leads to distress or impairment.

The wording on impairment is slightly different in the two classification schemes with DSMIV specifying 'impairment in social, occupational or other important areas of functioning' and ICD10 requiring that there is 'personal distress, or adverse impact on the social environment, or both, clearly attributable to the behaviour'.

Both ICD10 and DSMIV require that the pattern of behaviour is stable, and that the onset can be traced back to adolescent or early adult life. Again, both schemes have similar exclusion clauses, whereby the pattern of behaviour is not better accounted for or results from another mental disorder or can be explained by physical illness or drug use.

DSMIV divides personality disorders into three groups, clusters A, B and C. Although this is not done in ICD10, the categories of personality disorder are similar overall. The DSMIV clusters, their main characteristics, the cluster members and the ICD10 equivalents are summarized in table 9.3.

As we see, the specifics of the diagnostic terms and categories are similar in DSMIV and ICD10 systems. The main differences are that schizotypal disorder is classified as a mental disorder in F3, with schizophrenia and delusional disorders in ICD10, while in DSMIV, the disorder is included in Axis II with other personality disorders. Another important difference is that ICD10 does not recognize the existence of *narcissistic* personality disorder, and introduces a category, *emotionally unstable* personality disorder, *impulsive* type, that is not found in DSMIV. DSMIV on the other hand includes a rather broader concept of borderline personality disorder, something that ICD10 classifies as a particular subtype of emotionally unstable personality disorder. Elsewhere, the differences are largely in terminology rather than substance, in that ICD10 uses the term *anxious-avoidant*

Table 9.3. A summary of the DSMIV and ICD10 classification of personality disorders.

Cluster	Characteristics	DSMIV personality disorders	ICD10 equivalent personality disorder
A	Paranoid: persecutory beliefs, self reference, socially aloof or tending to mistake fantasy for reality	Paranoid Schizoid Schizotypal	Paranoid Schizoid
B	Antisocial: disruptive, aggressive, compulsive and histrionic behaviours	Antisocial Borderline Histrionic Narcissistic	Dissocial Emotionally unstable Borderline type Impulsive type Histrionic
C	Anxious/avoidant: high levels of anxiety, fearfulness, dependency or obsessionality	Avoidant Dependent Obsessive compulsive	Anxious Dependent Anankastic

personality disorder where DSMIV uses the term *avoidant* personality disorder and ICD10 uses the term *anankastic* to describe *obsessive-compulsive* personality disorder.

Detecting and measuring personality disorder

Despite this apparently high level of convergence of the two main current classifications, there is less overall agreement about how best to measure personality disorder. As with diagnostic interviews, primarily concerned with mental disorders (Axis I conditions according to DSMIV), some instruments proceed in a 'top down' fashion, being designed specifically to arrive at a diagnosis of personality disorder in a way that is governed by the structure of the criteria, whereas others proceed in a 'bottom up' fashion, aiming, in the first instance, to define component behaviours. There is also a difficulty in that most studies find that most categories of personality disorder are not usually found in 'pure culture', but rather individuals who fulfil the general criteria for having a personality disorder also tend to fulfil the criteria for more than one specific category.

The approaches that are used to measure and classified personality disorder can be divided into three groups.

1 Self-report questionnaires. As with measurement of personality in the normal range these are usually in the form of a series of 'yes/no' items.
2 Structured or semi-structured interviews. These are administered face-to-face with the subjects and, in general, the interviewer requires some degree of training.
3 Informant based instruments. These are measures that are based upon the reports of an informant other than the subject themselves.

Also, in addition to instruments for measuring personality disorder as a whole, some instruments concentrate on attempting to assess a particular category of personality disorder. The most common disorder-specific measures are for antisocial personality and schizotypal personality.

We will first look at instruments for measuring and classifying personality disorder in general. These are summarized in table 9.4. The Minnesota Multiphasic Personality Inventory (MMPI) is the oldest instrument still in current use, having been available for more than half a century. It is now commonly the second edition the MMPI-2 that is used in clinical practice and research. The MMPI was originally designed to assess psychopathology generally, and the basic method of construction was to contrast the responses of healthy controls with criterion groups of patients suffering from a variety of disorders or subjects judged clinically to be at an extreme on a particular trait. The 'clinical scales' in the MMPI-2 are *hypochondriasis, depression, hysteria, psychopathic deviate, masculinity-feminity, paranoia, psychasthenia, schizophrenia, hypomania* and *social introversion*. Despite its very widespread use the MMPI has been criticized for lacking a consistent measurement model, having a heterogenous scale content, having overlapping scales and having 'suspect' published norms (Helmes and Reddon 1993). It also has the drawback of using diagnostic concepts that are not closely in keeping with the current orthodoxies of DSM and ICD, so that it tends to give only low to moderate levels of agreement with DSM based interviews such as the SCID-II (Hills 1995). Nevertheless, it could be argued that the MMPI has withstood careful scrutiny of its biological validity as a personality measure, in that twin studies have shown that its clinical scales have moderate heritability and that there are genetic influences on both profile elevation and shape (DiLalla *et al.* 1996).

Table 9.4. Instruments for measuring and classifying personality disorder.

Instrument	Author (s)	Method	Diagnostic criteria	Approximate time complete
Minnesota Multiphasic Personality Inventory (MMPI and MMPI-2)	Hathaway and McKinley 1967, Butcher 1990	Self report	10 'clinical scales' (see text)	30 minutes
International Personality Disorder Examination (IPDE)	Loranger et al. 1994	Semi-structured interview with subject	ICD 10, DSMIIIR	1–2 hours
Personality Assessment Schedule (PAS)	Tyrer et al. 1984	Semi-structured interview with informant	DSMIIIR	1 hour
Structured Interview for DSMIII Personality Disorders (SIPD)	Stangl et al. 1985	Structured interview with subject	DSMIII	>1 hour
Standardized Assessment of Personality (SAP)	Pilgrim and Mann 1990	Semi-structured interview with informant	ICD 10, DSMIIIR	15 minutes
Personality Disorder Questionnaire – Revised (PDQ-R)	Hyler et al. 1992	Self report by subject or informant report	DSMIIIR	30 minutes
Screening Test for Comorbid Personality Disorders (STCPD)	Dowson 1992	Self report by subject or informant report	DSMIIIR	10–15 minutes
Structured Clinical Interview for DSM IIIR Personality Disorders (SCID-II)	Spitzer et al. 1992	Interview with subject	DSMIIIR	60–90 minutes

As we see in table 9.4, most of the other instruments are designed to arrive at DSMIII or DSMIIIR criteria. (At the time of writing, only two have yet been published in an updated DSMIV edition, but the differences between DSMIII, DSMIIIR and DSMIV are comparatively small with respect to personality disorder). Some instruments also allow the interviewer to arrive at a diagnosis using ICD10 criteria. That apart, there is a big range in the time taken to complete the assessment, from ten minutes up to two hours. Some instruments are designed for use only with subjects themselves, while others require independent information from an informant. Apart from the MMPI the questionnaire measures can be completed either by the subject or an informant or both. The Personality Disorder Questionnaire-Revised (PDQ-R) (Hyler *et al.* 1992) is particularly thorough. It has the virtue of covering every component required to make a DSMIIIR diagnosis of personality disorder and consists of 152 questions. The STCPD (Dowson 1992) is a screening questionnaire that contains a smaller number of PDQ-R type items in a modified format to improve acceptability (see below).

Like the PDQ-R, most of the instruments listed in the table were explicitly devised to arrive at preset diagnostic criteria so that they are essentially 'top down' in structure. That is, unlike some of the interviews that are used to make a classification of psychiatric disorders generally (see chapter 5), these instruments used for detecting personality disorder have not been constructed in 'bottom up' fashion, where the starting point is the component items or symptoms. Having said that, the longer interviews, the International Personality Disorder Examination (IPDE) (Loranger *et al.* 1994) and the Structured Clinical Interview for DSMIIIR Personality Disorders (SCID-II) (Spitzer *et al.* 1992) (see also appendix for website details) allow detailed probing of the symptoms of personality disorder. The IPDE is particularly thorough. Over 150 items are covered and the interviewer is required to ask the subject for examples or brief anecdotes to order to facilitate rating. Each is scored 0 if absent, 1 if probably and 2 if definitely present. The SCID-II, the IPDE and the PAS all require the interviewer to explore the persistence of symptoms and ensure that they have been present at least since early adulthood. The most recent version of the SCID-II can be used in conjunction with a self-report questionnaire, which is given to the subject before interview. The interviewer can then focus on the sections of interview dealing with questionnaire-positive items, in order to shorten the interview duration (First *et al.* 1994).

The Personality Assessment Schedule (PAS) (Tyrer *et al.* 1984), the first version of which was published before the introduction of operational definitions of personality disorder in DSMIII (American Psychiatric Association 1980), hence it is much less driven by preset diagnostic criteria in the way that it is constructed. The same can be said of the Standardized Assessment of Personality (SAP). This is a briefer interview which can be carried out face to face, or over the telephone (Pilgrim and Mann 1990) and uses an informant nominated by the subject, rather than the subject him or herself. The informant must have known the subject for at least five years. The interview has an open style of questioning at the beginning, where the interviewer searches for the use of key words by the informant. For example key words applying to antisocial personality disorder are 'irresponsible', 'aggressive' and 'lacks guilt' and some key words regarding obsessive compulsive (anankastic) personality are 'perfectionistic', 'over conscientious' and 'stubborn'. Where key words are elicited these form the basis for a more detailed exploration of a category (or categories) of personality disorder. Where no key words appear personality disorder is assumed to be absent.

The choice of instrument

How then does a researcher make a choice of instrument for a study of personality disorders? The answer to the question depends to a considerable extent on who is the target population and upon the time and manpower resources that are available. Regarding the population to be studied, one needs to consider the acceptability of the instrument and the extent to which assessments might be influenced by response set. Another consideration is whether an interview is required or whether almost as much information can be achieved from a questionnaire, which is inherently less expensive and time consuming. Reliability needs to be considered, both inter-rater agreement where an interview has been used, and the test re-test reliability for both interviews and self-report questionnaires. The specificity and sensitivity of the instrument needs to be considered, as does the extent to which the results will be affected by comorbidity, for example the co-occurrence of an axis I disorder such as depression and a personality disorder. Finally one needs to consider whether the assessment results in a valid classification. One obvious method of validation is to test whether the instrument is in good agreement with clinical diagnoses (but this, as we shall see, is not without problems). Another desirable quality is discriminant validity, the extent to which two or more types of disorder can be cleanly separated.

Acceptability, response set, and 'faking good'

We have already discussed the problems of response set in the context of questionnaires designed to measure normal personality. An attempt to avoid response set in assessing personality disorder is particularly important when it comes to the subject's view on acceptability of behaviours described in certain items. As we have noted, the PDQ-R is very comprehensive. However it consequently contains a range of questions that some respondents would find offensive, or which refer to characteristics that are transparently not socially desirable. There is therefore a risk that subjects will either deliberately or unconsciously give what they see as the 'correct' responses to questions rather that the responses that most accurately describe themselves.

This problem has been discussed by Dowson (1992), who has attempted to address it in a modified and shortened version of the PDQ-R called the Screening Test for Comorbid Personality Disorders (STCPD). An example relates to the DSMIIIR category of schizotypal personality disorder, where one of the features is 'Odd or eccentric behaviour or appearance, e.g. unkempt, unusual mannerisms, talks to self'. This is assessed in the PDQ-R by the asking the subject whether they agree with the statement 'People must think I'm pretty weird eccentric or strange'. This is modified in the STCPD to become 'People probably think that I am very different from other people because of my appearance, beliefs or the way I behave'. Dowson argues that this more tactful style of questioning when asking about odd or socially undesirable behaviour is useful in self-report versions of questionnaires, whereas in informants' versions such behaviours can be presented more directly. Even so, such modification can only go so far, and the STCPD still contains true/false items such as 'I have shoplifted', 'I have had sex with people I hardly know'.

Self-report or informant?

The issue of using slightly different wording in an informant versus a subject version of an instrument for measuring personality disorder leads to another question. Faced with a choice between informants or subjects themselves, who gives the better information? It could be argued that individuals with abnormal personalities are likely to be unreliable witnesses who, in addition to the potential problem of 'faking good', are not skilful at self reflection or at accurately reporting their social interactions. Informants who know the subject well may be more objective and dispassionate but on the other hand just the opposite may be true, and relatives might have deep-seated biases regarding someone they have labelled as the family's black sheep. Additionally informants, however well they know the subject, are likely to have some gaps in their biographical knowledge.

Clearly the ideal situation is to obtain data from both the subject and an informant but this may not always be feasible or practical and, as we have noted, some instruments come in only one version, only subject focused or only based on the informant's account. There is evidence that subjects themselves give *more* information. For example Dowson (1992) found that where positive PDQ-R responses were added up to give a score, self-reports gave significantly higher scores than informant report. This may reflect the simple fact that subjects had more knowledge of their own past lives than did informants. Indeed the agreement between subject and informant reports was highest for personality disorders involving more overt forms of behaviour, such as antisocial or schizotypal personalities. However in a proportion of subjects the informant derived score was substantially higher than that from the subject's own report, and the author suggested that such under reporting was associated with more severe personality problems.

A comparison between informant based interview, the SAP and a patient based interview the IPDE, has been carried out by Mann and colleagues (Mann *et al.* 1999). Interestingly, in view of the fact that most of the development of personality disorder questionnaires and interviews had hitherto been carried out in English speaking countries, mainly the US and the UK, the SAP/IPDE comparison was performed in Bangalore, India. Unfortunately the overall agreement between the two interviews in detecting ICD10 personality disorder was modest, with a kappa coefficient of 0.4. This is in keeping with an earlier comparison of patient based and informant based interviews in the US (Zimmerman *et al.* 1986). The best agreement in the Bangalore study was for dependent personality (kappa = 0.66) and the poorest was for dissocial personality (kappa = 0.09). However the authors found that if they accepted the findings of the longer and more detailed interview, the IPDE, as the 'gold standard' then the SAP proved to have a very high negative predictive value of 97%. That is the SAP, based on accounts from relatives or friends, failed to identify just 1 of 26 subjects classified as having an ICD10 personality disorder following an IPDE interview. Mann and colleagues have therefore proposed that, for purposes of epidemiological studies, a two-stage approach is desirable (see also chapter 7), where stage one uses the short informant based interview and stage two consists of the longer interview with subjects who are identified at stage one.

Reliability of the classification of personality disorder

All of the interviews listed in table 9.4 are reported by their authors to give good inter-rater agreement and importantly for informant-based interviews, the PAS and the SAP, inter-informant reliability is remarkably high (Mann *et al.* 1999). Given that one of the characteristics of personality disorders is they are enduring, the question of test re-test reliability is vital. All of the interviews in table 9.4 again are satisfactory in this respect (Tyrer 1990). However these instrument have in general been developed and standardized on psychiatric in- patients or outpatients, so the issue of how well they would perform in epidemiological studies is largely unknown (Zimmerman 1994). However a study of the SCID-II found good test re-test agreement in psychiatric settings but poorer stability in non-patient samples (First *et al.* 1994).

Of the questionnaire measures, the PDQ-R has been the most closely studied and shows high test re-test stability, as well as good internal consistency (Hyler *et al.* 1992). However it is worth noting that questionnaire measures in general have a tendency to identify more subjects as personality disordered than do interviews, and we will return to this in considering validity.

Specificity, comorbidity, and validity

A recurrent finding in studies using any of the standard instruments to define ICD10 or DSM IIIR criteria is that the majority of subjects detected as being cases of personality disorder, fulfil the criteria for not just one but for several categories of disorder. That is, comorbidity is the rule rather than the exception, and specificity in the sense of the ability to define and identify cases of a particular category of disorder in pure form is low. For example, a review of four studies found that the average proportion of subjects diagnosed as having multiple disorders was 85% (Widiger *et al.* 1988). The ability of a diagnostic process to categorize subjects into discrete and non-overlapping classes is also sometimes called discriminant validity. Clearly this is low if most subjects are given multiple diagnoses, but this leaves us with the question of whether there is a fundamental flaw in the diagnostic systems or whether we are dealing with disorders that in some senses are distinct but nevertheless really do cluster together. Attempts to examine this issue using multivariate statistical methods (e.g. Dowson 1992) have tended to find that only antisocial personality forms a relatively homogenous group. As discussed particularly in chapter 3 but also elsewhere throughout this book, the problem of comorbidity in psychiatric disorders is a recurrent one where modern non-hierarchical definitions of disorders are employed.

A rather different approach to determining validity is to compare the findings from structured interviews or questionnaires with the diagnoses of experienced clinicians. However this presupposes that the clinicians' diagnoses themselves have some inherent validity. Hyler and colleagues (1992) compared the diagnoses obtained using the Personality Diagnostic Questionnaire (PDQ) and subsequently the PDQ-R with clinical diagnoses. Although they found that a high questionnaire score was a useful general predictor of whether or not subjects had a clinically diagnosed personality disorder, there was a poor agreement overall with regard to specific categories. Only borderline personality showed reasonable agreement (kappa = 0.46) between the questionnaire derived and the clinical diagnosis. The authors postulated that the problems lay with failings of self-reports and the tendency for the questionnaire approach to 'over-diagnose'. However, as the test of over diagnosis was clinical judgement and we know that clinicians tend to have idiosyncratic and inconsistent approaches to diagnosing personality disorder, this conclusion can be called into question. In fact, in a study elsewhere that compared 'best estimate' consensus diagnoses assigned by a panel of clinicians with the diagnosis of personality disorder according to two structured interviews, the Personality Disorder Examination, (PDE) and the SIDP-R, the agreement was again poor with kappa coefficients below 0.4 (Pilkonis *et al.* 1995).

Instruments designed to measure and detect specific forms of personality disorder

The two types of personality deviation that have attracted specific attention are antisocial personality and schizotypy or schizotypal disorder. (As we noted earlier, schizotypal disorder is bracketed along with schizophrenia and other psychoses in the ICD10 classification, but here we follow the

DSMIII/DSMIV convention and approach it as a personality disorder or dimension).

Antisocial personality disorder

This has largely been a focus of research for those investigators whose aim is to predict disruptive or violent behaviour, particularly in forensic settings. Various instruments have been devised, mostly in North America, and among the most widely used to predict violence are the Dangerous Behavior Rating Scale (DBRS) (Menzies *et al.* 1985), the Violence Risk Appraisal Guide (VRAG) (Harris *et al.* 1993) and the Historical/Clinical Risk Management twenty item scale (HCR-20) (Webster *et al.* 1997). The VRAG and the HCR-20 contain a section to assess antisocial behaviour or 'psychopathy', based on the Psychopathy Checklist – Revised (PCL-R) (Hare 1991). The PCL-R, as its title suggests, consists of a checklist of items that is scored by the clinician or researcher on the basis of a combination of the best available information. It is therefore neither a structured interview nor a self-report questionnaire, but a clinical checklist. (It is therefore somewhat akin to, if much briefer than, checklists used elsewhere in research on psychopathology, such as OPCRIT [chapter 6]).

Although it contains several items that appear to depend on rather subjective judgements on the part of the rater (e.g. 'lacks empathy'), the PCL-R, its predecessor the Psychopathy Checklist (PCL) and tools that include their items such as the HCR-20, generally have been shown to be moderate to good predictors of violence or disruptive behaviour in psychiatric clinical or forensic settings (Dolan and Doyle 2000). A shortened version of the PCL-R, the PCL-SV (Hart *et al.* 1995) appears to be almost as useful. The PCL-R is said to have a stable factor structure (Hare 1991) with two main dimensions reflecting interpersonal/affective traits and 'psychopathic' behaviour. In the PCL-SV the items describing interpersonal and affective characteristics are:

- Superficial
- Grandiose
- Manipulative
- Lacks remorse
- Lacks empathy
- Does not accept responsibility

The items describing psychopathic behaviour are:

- Impulsive
- Poor behaviour controls
- Lacks goals
- Irresponsible
- Adolescent antisocial behaviour
- Adult antisocial behaviour

Each of the items on the PCL-SV is scored on a 0–2 scale giving a possible maximum total score of 20. Typically researchers have taken cut-offs where, for example a score of 18 or more denotes definite psychopathy, and a score or 12 or more suggests a high risk of violence (Dolan and Doyle 2000).

Schizotypal personality disorder

This is a comparatively recently introduce category. Meehl (1962) first coined the term schizotypy to describe the 'sub clinical' features of those close relatives of schizophrenics who, while not showing the full-blown disorder themselves, had various symptoms reflecting a schizophrenic diathesis or susceptibility. Subsequently twin and adoption studies of schizophrenia published during the 1960s and 1970s highlighted a range of abnormalities or personality traits that did indeed appear to have a genetic relationship to schizophrenia (McGuffin *et al.* 1995). These came to be called 'schizophrenia spectrum disorders' or, in DSMIII, (American Psychiatric Association 1980) schizotypal personality disorder. The main components of DSM III schizotypal personality disorder remain unchanged in DSMIV and form the basis of the ICD10 category of schizotypal disorder. The symptoms include unusual beliefs that amount to over valued ideas rather than frank delusions (see chapter 2) and perceptual distortions rather than overt hallucinations. The main categories of schizotypal symptoms are:

- Ideas of reference
- Paranoid thinking
- Magical thinking
- Recurrent illusions
- Social anxiety
- Social isolation

There are also features about which the individual is unlikely to complain and which are in effect schizotypal signs rather than symptoms. They are:

- Odd behaviour
- Odd speech patterns
- Poor rapport
- Aloofness/coldness

Therefore in order to fully assess schizotypal disorder one needs to have either observer ratings from a clinician, or reports from informants in addition to self-reported symptoms. Two structured interviews have been specifically devised to assess schizotypal personality, the Schedule for Schizotypal Personalities (SSP) (Baron *et al.* 1981) and the Structured Interview for Schizotypy (Kendler *et al.* 1989). Both seem to have utility and validity in respect of being capable of detecting increased rates of schizotypy in the relatives of schizophrenics. However, as elsewhere, questionnaire measures offer the potential advantages of being quicker and less expensive. In addition, particularly with a potentially sensitive group of subjects, questionnaires may be less intrusive than interviews. A number of questionnaire measures have been devised to measure schizotypy of which the Kings Schizotypy Questionnaire (KSQ) (Williams 1993, Jones *et al.* 2000) is among the most recent. The KSQ contains just the symptom component of schizotypy incorporated into a 63 item scale of yes/no questions. It has been shown to have good psychometric properties with high internal consistency (Cronbach's alpha = 0.81) and good test re-test reliability (r = 0.73). It also was initially shown to have its highest scores in schizophrenic patients, and intermediate scores in their relatives at a level that was significantly higher than controls (Williams 1993). Unfortunately an attempt at replication of this pattern confirmed the patient/control difference but found that the KSQ score in schizophrenics' relatives was slightly lower than than in the controls. This may have been because 'defensive' responses to the KSQ in relatives or have been a result of a high (52%) refusal rate in the relatives so that it is possible that the responders were a self selected, low schizotypy group. However a failure to detect increased schizotypy levels in the relatives of schizophrenics has occurred in a number of other questionnaire based studies (eg Maier *et al.* 1994) which raises a question mark over the general usefulness of the approach.

Discrete disorders or extremes on continua?

The question of whether psychopathology is better measured and described dimensionally than categorically has been a recurrent theme throughout much of this volume, but nowhere is the issue more pressing than in the case of personality disorder. This is so because dimensional approaches are now universally accepted as the better and more useful way of describing normal personality, whereas categorical approaches remain the dominant and officially sanctioned way of describing personality disorder, despite widespread dissatisfaction with the current classification schemes. Not long after the introduction of DSMIII, Frances (1982) defended the categorical method in personality diagnosis, pointing out that there are many things in nature that are better viewed categorically, even if this does not capture the total reality or reliably distinguish subtle shades of difference. Colour variation is a good example of a phenomenon that we know results from continuous variation within the visible spectrum but where nevertheless referring to colours as distinct named categories is 'quite handy when one wants to buy a suit or describe a sunset' (Frances 1982). On the other hand for some tasks involving light waves, such as a study of refraction, a dimensional system is more precise and contains more information. The argument then is that for everyday purposes categories win out because they are 'simple and convenient abstractions of what is essential'.

If this is accepted we also need to accept a related caveat. The methods used in defining categories of personality disorder are dependent on *proto-types*. That is, each description of a personality type represents an idealized 'typical' case, but in real life real cases are rarely more than approximations to that prototype. Frances (1982) has argued that again this is not peculiar to the classification of different forms of psychopathology. In fact most categories in most areas of biology turn out to be probabilistic rather than fulfilling the ideal of being homogenous, mutually exclusive and jointly exhaustive (Kendell 1975). The principal argument therefore in favour of categories to describe personality disorder is essentially the same as that in other areas of psychopathology (and see also chapter 1), other areas of science and indeed other areas of life; categories have greater utility and are easier to handle than dimensions.

The counter argument is that categories are indeed often handy but their utility in the sphere of personality disorder is in doubt. The reliability, even using operational definitions, is low, most cases fulfil criteria for more than one category and in contrast to axis I disorders, a diagnosis of personality disorder does not provide a useful indicator of how a patient is best treated. There is also a problem that is common to operationally defined categories generally, that the cut-offs for the presence or absence of a disorder may be arbitrary (see also chapter 3). Widiger (1993) for example, has pointed out that the thresholds for nine out of eleven DSMIIIR categories of personality disorder were simply decided by a panel of experts, unguided by any data. This leads to clinical conundrums such as how to classify someone who has only four rather than the required five (out of a possible nine) symptoms of compulsive personality disorder. Even if they are impaired by their four symptoms, is it reasonable that they are simply classified as having no disorder? In contrast there are reliable and valid dimensional methods of describing and measuring personality, so why not extend the use of these approaches to the study of those who probably differ only quantitatively, not qualitatively from normal?

In fact attempts to tackle personality disorder using dimensional approaches are not new. We have earlier briefly discussed the use of the MMPI, which effectively consists of a set of diagnostic categories reformulated as symptom scales. A patient who completes the MMPI can then be assigned a profile on a set of scales rather than a single diagnosis. Eysenck (1960) proposed an even more radical departure from standard clinical classification. He suggested that personality disordered subjects could be 'mapped' dimensionally using E and N scales. Thus psychopathic and hysterical personalities would be characterized by high neuroticism and high extraversion. Obsessional or anxious/avoidant personality types would also score highly on neuroticism but would typically be low on extraversion. More recent attempts to explore EPQ dimensions in relation to personality disorder have produced interesting, if not entirely clear cut results. For example Deary *et al.* (1998) carried out principal components analysis and confirmatory factor analysis on a large sample of university undergraduates who had completed DSMIIIR personality disorder questionnaires and the EPQ. They found four broad factors (rather than three clusters as proposed by the authors of DSMIIIR). These were an asthenic factor related to neuroticism, an antisocial factor associated with psychoticism, an asocial factor relating to extraversion-introversion and an anankastic factor.

There has also been considerable recent interest in reformulating psychopathy (Widiger and Lynam 1998) or personality disorders generally in terms of a five-factor model. There is reasonable agreement among theorists about what would be the expected patterns of score for extraversion and neuroticism (which are largely in keeping with Eysenck's original

Table 9.5. The predicted relationship between Big Five dimensions and DSM personality disorder clusters.

Dimension	Cluster		
	A (paranoid)	B (antisocial)	C (anxious avoidant)
Extraversion	−	+	−
Neuroticism	+	+	+
Agreeableness	−	−	+
Conscientiousness	?	−	+
Openness	?	+/?	−/?

+ = high scores, − = low scores, ? = no clear prediction

speculations) and to a lesser extent there is a consensus on the role of agreeableness and conscientiousness. However, the place of openness to experience is less clear. The predicted pattern of scores for the three main DSMIV clusters of personality type is shown in table 9.5.

As we have noted, the personality dimensions proposed by Cloninger (1987) were aimed at providing 'a systematic method for clinical description and classification' and the author has made explicit attempts to relate his personality measures to psychopathology. The broad predicted relationship between DSMIV personality disorder clusters and three of Cloninger's dimensions, novelty seeking, harm avoidance and award dependence, are summarized in table 9.6.

Unfortunately it is too early to arrive at firm conclusions about the usefulness of either the Big Five or Cloninger's approaches to assessing personality disorder within a DSM type framework. From a Big Five perspective, the empirical evidence is somewhat confusing. One reviewer finds reasonable

Table 9.6. The predicted relationship between 3 of Cloninger's dimensions and DSM personality disorder clusters.

Dimension	Cluster		
	A (paranoid)	B (antisocial)	C (anxious avoidant)
Novelty seeking	−	+	−
Harm avoidance	−	−	+
Reward dependence	−	−	+

+ = high scores, − = low scores

agreement between studies but notes that inconsistencies have probably arisen because of differences in instruments (rather than broad concepts) and because insufficient attention has been paid to peer ratings compared with self reports (Dyce 1997). Others (e.g. Yeung *et al.* 1993) have found only a modest relationship between Big Five dimensions and personality disorder types or have found a lack of specificity in the pattern of scores (Morey *et al.* 2000). That is, personality disorder can be distinguished form normal personality but there is poor discrimination between DSM categories. Of course, research comparing categories and dimensions may simply be producing confusing results because the current categories are inherently flawed, and we tend to agree with the advocates of dimensional models who argue that these need to be taken into account in the construction of future classifications in DSMV and ICD11.

CHAPTER 10

Psychopathology in the Twenty-first Century

Technological and clinical advances

Considerable progress in our understanding of mental disorders has taken place over the past few decades. In particular technological advances have come in the fields of functional and structural neuroimaging, pharmacology, and genetics, and important conceptual and experimental progress has been made in cognitive psychology. These, in turn, have increased the potential to unlock the secrets of the biological bases of psychiatric disorders and have encouraged those who aim to understand the interplay between biological substrate and environmental insult in the causation of psychological problems. For example, the combination of cognitive psychology and new developments in functional neuroimaging is beginning to provide valuable insights into how the brain processes information, and how this is altered in individuals with psychological disturbances and/or psychiatric disorder.

The revolution in molecular genetics has also provided enormous potential for insights into the biological bases of psychiatric disorder. We have known for many years that genes play a major role in a variety of psychiatric disorders, and with recent technological advances we now have the capability of identifying them (Plomin *et al.* 1997). The Human Genome Project has reached the stage of a nearly complete draft sequence, partially annotated, (International Human Genome Sequencing Consortium 2001, Venter *et al.* 2001) of the entire 4-nucleotide base structure of human DNA. Currently a collaboration between the medical research charity, the Wellcome Trust and several major pharmaceutical companies, the Single Nucleotide Polymorphism (SNP) Consortium is working to identify the variations in the nucleotide sequence that occur at approximately 1000 kilobase intervals throughout the genome. The majority of SNPs occur in noncoding regions and probably have no functional significance. Nevertheless they can be used as 'anonymous' markers to pinpoint the location of disease genes, as the first step towards identifying them in the process called positional cloning (see McGuffin and Martin 1999, for a brief introduction). Of even greater interest are SNPs occurring in coding or regulatory regions that alter function and are sources of individual differences in levels of gene expression or protein structure. Rapid throughput genotyping technologies now make it possible to do hundreds of genotypings in the time it used to take to do tens, and for around the same costs. Consequently it is becoming increasingly easy to analyse the large samples generated by linkage and association studies. Positional cloning approaches have already led to the identification of the genes involved in rare single gene psychiatric disorders such as Huntington's disease and early onset familial Alzheimer's disease, and are likely to lead on to the eventual identification of the multiple genes involved in more complex and common disorders (McGuffin *et al.* 2001).

However, identifying the biological underpinnings either from genetics or neuroimaging research will not provide all of the answers in understanding the development of psychiatric disorders. External or environmental factors are also recognized as making significant contributions; indeed one of the most consistent findings from genetics studies of behaviour is that the environment has a significant role (Plomin *et al.* 1997). Carefully developed interview techniques for evaluating the impact of developmental adversity and significant life events, (Brown and Harris 1978, Bifulco *et al.* 2000) have led to an enhanced understanding of the role of environmental risk factors, as well as their interplay with familial and genetic factors (Farmer *et al.* 2000).

As well as the promise of major advances in understanding the aetiology of mental disorders, there have also been several national epidemiological studies undertaken in the 1980s and 1990s (Regier *et al.* 1993, Kessler *et al.* 1994, Jenkins *et al.* 1997). Although it can be argued that some of these have posed as many questions about the prevalence and incidence of psychiatric disorder as they have answered (Regier *et al.* 1998), they have provided important information for service planners. In addition, such studies have helped further understanding about the variation in prevalence and incidence of disorder in different geographic, socio-demographic and cultural settings.

We also enter the new millennium with much improved treatments for those suffering from mental disorders. These include 'cleaner' drugs with fewer disabling side effects, as well as clinically effective psychotherapies. The replacement of large, old and stigmatized mental hospitals with the delivery of treatment at or close to home, via community based teams, has been more acceptable to most sufferers from mental disorders. In addition, the stigma associated with having a mental disorder appears at last to be reducing (if slowly). This may in part be associated with more sensitive coverage in the media (Brindle 2000) (although this is still decidedly mixed). It also noteworthy that it is becoming more acceptable for famous personalities to 'come out', acknowledging that they have suffered from a mental disorder. For example, it has been widely reported that an ex-President of the United States has Alzheimer's disease, and a number of well-known show business personalities have openly discussed their problems with affective disorder or substance misuse. In association with the general acceptance that mental disorders have a partly biological basis, and are not just attributable due to 'weakness' or personality flaw, has come a determination that those with mental disorders should be personally involved with decision making. Alongside this there has been a growing advocacy movement and a trend toward using the terms 'user' or 'client' instead of 'patient', which some consider paternalistic or patronizing. (Interestingly there is some evidence, at least in the UK, that most users actually prefer to be called patients [Ritchie *et al.* 2000]). There might also be a hope that greater public awareness, lowered stigma and increased user involvement in the shape of services should be associated with improved access to high quality care. Unfortunately the story here is mixed, and there is little evidence in most western countries that the savings resulting from deinstitutionalization have been passed on to patients. In fact in the UK the proportion of total health spend that goes to mental health has decreased over the last three decades.

The improved methods for measuring psychopathology described in this book, despite their flaws, have certainly contributed to these advances in biological and psychosocial research, and arguably have contributed also to improvements in the treatment and quality of life for those with mental disorder. However, so far we have focused on benefits and advances, which only cover part of the picture. Many problems still remain, which we will now discuss.

Identifying phenotypes: searching for the causes of psychopathology

As we have already highlighted, two promising research fields for those currently involved in exploring the aetiology of mental disorders are genetics and neuroimaging. Both types of research seek to find differences (in genetic profile or in brain structure and function) between those with and without psychopathology or between different psychopathological groupings. Consequently, the main clinical requirement is a clear and reliable definition of the signs and symptoms. The issues that will need consideration in the future are much the same as in the past, and are as follows. First, there will be further changes to national and international nosologies, which will pose problems regarding comparability with earlier studies. Second, there is the question of whether there are major subdivisions within the main categories that are aetiologically significant, and thirdly, there is a need to continue the much-debated issue of categories versus dimensions.

Changes to national and international nosologies

The new DSMV and ICD11 classifications are being planned as this book is being written. As in all previous classifications, DSMV and ICD11, will only represent 'a set of hypotheses about reality, subject to change and development' (Robins and Helzer 1986). The regular review of these major nosologies will continue indefinitely, or at least for as long as the validity of their definitions remains in doubt. As Spitzer and colleagues stated in 1975;

> Premature closure (of a diagnostic schema) can be avoided only by the recognition that any classification system and its criteria should be regarded with varying degrees of tentativeness and should be subject to continual revision

according to new knowledge . . . Perhaps the true value of the suggested criteria will be demonstrated, not by how long they remain unchanged, but by the rapidity with which they facilitate research that results in their modification and improvement.

This suggests that the problems associated with all previous changes of major nosologies will also pertain to DSMV and ICD11, and to future classifications of mental disorders. These we have outlined in chapter 6. One of the main problems relates to the fact that seemingly minor changes to individual items within the operational definition can have a significant impact on the numbers of subjects defined as cases (Farmer *et al.* 1993). We have discussed this problem in some detail in chapter 6 in relation to operational criteria for schizophrenia (Farmer *et al.* 1993). Small changes relating to one item on the 'impairment' associated with the disorder, has led to quite a marked impact on the number of subjects diagnosed according to DSMIIIR criteria, compared to DSMIII. Definitional changes have similarly led to an apparent increase in personality disorder in the United States (Widiger 1993).

We have also showed that the method of selecting subjects has a major impact on the proportion of cases diagnosed according a particular definition. Older subjects, who have passed through the period of risk, are more likely to be diagnosed as cases than younger acutely admitted subjects, who will have had much shorter histories. Similarly, there are also issues relating to how the diagnostic information is collected. Different diagnostic interviews e.g. SCAN and SADS-L can also give rather different diagnostic profiles, even when the same clinicians give each interview to the same subjects (Farmer *et al.* 1993).

In addition, such regular changes in the boundaries of disorder with successive classifications could mean that those defined as having a disorder now are very different from those thus defined in the past. However, some reassurance that this is not the case, at least for psychotic disorders, is provided in a study by Jablensky and colleagues (1993). These authors applied modern operational definitions to the detailed case descriptions, from Kraepelin's original research (Jablensky *et al.* 1993), using the Present State Examination syndrome checklist (Wing *et al.* 1974). The authors found that the overall concordance between Kraepelin's original diagnoses and computer assisted ICD9 diagnoses was 88.6%. They concluded that the diagnosis of dementia praecox in 1908 and ICD9 schizophrenia of the 1970s referred to the same syndrome (Jablensky 1997).

Indeed Jablensky and colleagues (1993) state that it is somewhat surprising that the Kraepelinian dichotomy, as the fundamental conceptual framework within which research in the psychoses has been conducted, has not changed. This is despite many doubts by researchers and clinicians as well as many attempts at alternative formulations.Elsewhere, the author has commented that this is because

> The conceptual model of the pathogenesis of schizophrenia and affective psychosis proposed by Kraepelin, is consonant with present day ideas arising out of neuroscience and genetics ... the lesson to be drawn is that the nosological argument could be put on hold until basic understanding is gained of the specific mechanisms of syndromogenesis across diagnostic boundaries. (Jablensky 1997)

This issue, which exercised researchers at the turn of the twentieth century, remains just as pertinent today, and is likely remain with us for the foreseeable future.

Heterogeneity of diagnostic categories

Another major issue relates to the phenotypic heterogeneity of the majority of diagnostic categories, and whether any sub-typology has aetiological significance. In other words, does the observed phenotypic variation in signs and symptoms between individuals defined as having the same disorder reflect underlying aetiological differences which may indicate, for example, different responses to treatment. This has been described (McGuffin *et al.* 1987) as the 'one from many', or 'many from one' issue. For example, swelling of the feet and legs (oedema) can be caused by many disorders including heart disease or kidney failure. Consequently the same syndrome, oedema, requires different treatment depending on the underlying cause. In contrast, infection with Trepomena pallidum causes syphilis, a disease with many physical manifestations (the 'great mimic'), including genital sores, rashes, and later damage to certain tract of nerves in the spinal column and to the cerebral hemispheres. This is an example of the 'many (syndromes) from one (cause)'. In this example, early treatment with penicillin cures or prevents all of the syndromes caused by the infection.

The failures to find significant differences on various measures (e.g. brain structure or function) between those with and those without the main psychiatric disorders has led to some frustration. Few differences have been found, and those that have, have seldom been replicated. This has led some researchers to turn their attentions instead to try to find differences between various subgroups of a disorder. In particular, schizophrenia has been variously subdivided and each successive generation of researchers has produced yet another sub-typology (Lorr *et al.* 1963, Farmer *et al.* 1985, Liddle 1987, Nakaya *et al.* 1999). The main reason that these efforts focus on schizophrenia is that the original work by Kraepelin and colleagues, in defining the syndrome, drew together various individual syndromal descriptions under the umbrella term dementia praecox (see chapter 1). Subsequently, the concept of different syndromes constituting subtypes of schizophrenia has been kept going for over 100 years. However, the advent of computer technology in the 1980s facilitated the application of sophisticated statistical methods to explore sub-typing. Consequently, schizophrenic symptoms and signs have been subjected to such approaches as factor analysis, cluster analysis, and discriminant function analysis, to try and identify meaningful symptom/sign complexes (factor analysis) or groupings of subjects (cluster analysis). Such sub-typing efforts have lead to much debate, although some have concluded that methodological inconsistencies have caused many artefacts (Stuart *et al.* 1999).

The majority of sub-typologies have not been validated against an external criterion, and this remains their main limitation. Also, to date no sub-typology has shown any replicable differences which have aetiological significance. Rather than producing meaningful new categories, 'carving nature at the joints', attempts to subtype schizophrenia are more akin to slicing salami (McGuffin *et al.* 1987). No doubt there will continue to be attempts to find the natural divisions both between and within disorders in the future. Rather than the production of yet more sub-typologies, one of the more helpful 'spin offs', from the application of multivariate statistical approaches, is that they facilitate the derivation of *factors scores*, which can be used as dimensions.

Dimensions versus categories revisited

In the previous chapter we compared dimensional and categorical approaches to personality and personality disorder, but the general theme has been a recurrent one throughout this book. Indeed, as we have discussed in chapter 3, one of the original premises upon which operational definitions were first devised in psychiatry, was that of thresholds being imposed on dimensions. According to Hempel's (1961) original proposal, the process of defining operationally should include the detection of each of the components, symptoms or signs 'X', and answering the question 'does the subject exhibit this much of X?'. Most psychopathological symptoms can be quantified, indeed symptoms like low mood or anxiety can be readily conceptualized as dimensions. Even symptoms that appear to be clear dichotomies (present or absent), such as delusional beliefs can be quantified. For example, a score can be devised according to how strongly the belief is held, or whether there is any element of doubt. Another way of scoring might be according to whether the beliefs dominate the thoughts and behaviour of an individual, or whether he or she can turn attention to other matters and behave with apparent normality.

The importance of the diagnostic process has been discussed in chapter 1. However, some researchers have argued against confining research to just the examination of diagnostic categories, and that research on symptoms may be more fruitful than research on syndromes (Costello 1992). The main reasons for this, cited by Costello, are (i) the questionable validity of psychiatric diagnostic systems, (ii) the requirement to assess large number of different types of symptom rather than adequately measure individual items, (iii) whether there is a true cut off between a psychiatric syndrome and normality, and (iv) the problems of overlapping of symptoms between diagnostic groups.

Persons (1986) explained this last problem in the following way. If a researcher wishes to examine the possible biological correlates of schizophrenic formal thought disorder he or she may consider that the mechanism is present in subjects with schizophrenia and absent in those who do not have the disorder. However this research strategy is unlikely to be successful for the following reasons (Persons 1986). First, not all people with schizophrenia exhibit thought disorder, although some do. Second, even those who do experience the symptom do not experience it all the time and may not be thought disordered when tested. Third, individuals with other disorders such as bipolar disorder may also experience formal thought disorder (Harvey and Neale 1983).

Costello (1992) argues that although the pursuit of valid psychiatric syndromes must continue, more research time should be spent on the investigation of specific symptoms and their interrelationships. In contrast, Mojtabai and Rieder (1998) have posed a counter argument. These authors found little evidence in support of the thesis that (i) symptoms have higher reliability and validity compared to diagnostic categories, (ii) that underlying pathological mechanisms are symptom specific and (iii) that elucidation of the process of symptom development will lead to the discovery of the causes of syndromes.

Important points have been made on both sides of this argument. For many types of research, it is probably necessary to both rate *disorder* as well as adopt a *dimensional approach* to measuring psychopathology. For example, much molecular genetic research now focuses on quantitative traits, since most trait or disorders associated with psychiatry, are both multi-factorial and polygenic i.e. more than a few genes are involved. Consequently genetic studies of common disorders are concerned with identifying 'quantitative trait loci' or QTLs. In chapter 6 we have described the use of polydiagnostic systems such as the OPCRIT checklist and how this facilitates the application of multiple different operational definitions of a disorder. Most of the individual items from OPCRIT incorporate either severity or duration ratings, and these can also be employed separately as a quantitative measure (Farmer *et al.* 1985). Similarly, the structured interviews described in chapter 5 can also provide a source of carefully rated individual items of psychopathology that do not have be examined according to a particular diagnosis, but can also be considered quantitatively. For example, the items rated at interview can be summated, to provide a dimensional score. We have also described the use of threshold scores to provide 'cut-off' points, (case / not a case) as well as summating scores to provide a dimension for a number of the rating scales described in chapter 7. Much of the research currently being undertaken into the aetiology of schizophrenia includes both a diagnostic interview with additional dimensional ratings of different (positive and negative) symptom groups, for example, using the Positive and Negative Symptom Scale (PANSS) (Kay *et al.* 1991).

Most of our discussion so far has related to searches for causes of psychopathology. We would argue that discovering more about aetiology will be the key issue in improving classification and diagnosis. Once causes are identified, our current diagnostic conventions can be modified, but improved treatments for those with mental disorders are also promised. Arguably, more immediate problems for those with psychopathology and their relatives relate to political and health care planning. These issues are associated with case finding and health services research.

Finding cases: future issues for epidemiological and primary care research

Two recent major epidemiological studies in US have come to rather different conclusions about the prevalence of psychiatric disorders. The

Epidemiological Catchment Area (ECA) study (Regier *et al.* 1993, and see also chapter 3) was undertaken between 1980 and 1985, and found lifetime prevalence rates for any psychiatric disorder of between 32% and 44%. In contrast, the National Comorbidity Study (NCS), undertaken in the early 1990s at the request of the National Institutes of Mental Health in the US as a partial replication of the ECA study (Kessler *et al.* 1994), found lifetime prevalence rates for 'any disorder' of 48%. The NCS also found higher co-morbidity rates for depression and anxiety compared to the ECA study. In addition, 29% of NCA subjects, compared with only 20% of ECA participants, met diagnostic criteria for at least one disorder 'within the past year'.

The discrepant findings between these two ostensibly similar studies suggested that further work on the standardization of the methods for measuring psychopathology is required. According to Regier and colleagues (1998) this standardization is required in order to (i) reduce the apparent discrepancies in prevalence rates between similar population surveys (Regier *et al.* 1993, Kessler *et al.* 1994) (ii) differentiate clinically significant severity from less severe self limiting morbidity. We have already pointed out that slight changes to individual items, coding algorithms or combinatorial rules can make big differences to the number of subjects rated as 'cases' according to different operational definitions (Farmer *et al.* 1993 and see also chapter 6). Consequently, when a new DSM is produced, seemingly very modest changes to the operational definitions can lead to major changes in the number of individuals who are defined as having a disorder. This may well be one of the reasons for the discrepancy found between the ECA study, which applied DSMIII (American Psychiatric Association 1980) operational criteria and the NCS, where the DSMIIIR criteria (American Psychiatric Association 1987) were applied. The method of assessment e.g. face to face or telephone interview, as well as the structured interview employed to obtain the data could have also contributed to the discrepancies in prevalence, found in the two studies. Although both studies used related interviews (the ECA used the DIS, while the NCS used the CIDI), there are sufficient differences between the two for this to have an impact on overall prevalence estimates. As has been pointed out by Regier and colleagues (1998), these seemingly subtle differences between these two similar studies could affect political and health policy. As the authors state:

> Discrepant and/or high prevalence rates will have particular implications for determining treatment need in the context of managed care definitions of medical necessity ... it is reasonable to hypothesize that some syndromes in the

community represent transient homeostatic responses to internal or external stimuli that do not represent true psychopathologic disorder. Regier *et al.* 1998

In a further comment on the problems of defining clinical significance, Frances (1998) also asserted that future epidemiological studies should study fewer disorders and concentrate on those that are more severe and more likely to affect public health policy. He suggested that case definition should require measurable functional impairment as well as symptom evaluation.

These issues are also relevant for research into the psychiatric morbidity in primary care and similar populations. As we have mentioned in chapter 7, the presentation, distress and impairment associated with psychopathology in primary care and in those who are hospitalized for physical disorders is somewhat different to that seen by psychiatrists. Rating scales and diagnostic interviews that have greater relevance to these settings need to be devised, as well as measures of functioning and impairment. Such issues have been the focus of health services research.

New approaches to measuring psychopathology

The major changes in the way health services have been provided for those with mental disorders has led to the suggestion that there is a need for a new approach to measurement (Ustun 1997). This has been described as a need for a *paradigm shift*, in order to consider service utilization, need for care, treatment matching and outcome evaluation when measuring psychopathology (Ustun 1997). This author has gone on to say that 'A disablement construct may provide an important complementary prospective and insight for services research' (Ustun 1997). On a similar theme Jenkins has commented that 'We urgently need a nosology that will allow us to capture the various dimensions of positive mental health building on such concepts as life skills, loss of control, and coping strategies' (Jenkins 1997). There are already several rating scales and interviews that measure quality of life, global impairment of function, service utilization, treatment response and side effect profile. To some extent, these important aspects of global functioning are captured by the five axial system incorporated in the DSM classifications (American Psychiatric Association 1980, 1987, 1994). Certainly, in the research literature, most work has concentrated on axes 1 and 2; there being by comparison little interest in axes 3, 4 and 5 (see chapter 3). However, maybe it is time to take a new look at their application.

Another important political issue, particularly within the UK, has been risk assessment. High profile cases of homicide by those with psychopathology, has focused attention on the need to evaluate the risk for violence. Fortunately, the mentally disordered offender is rare among those who have psychopathology. In earlier studies, the best predictors of violence in those with psychopathology were found to be the same as for non-disordered offenders (Monahan 1994). However, more recently the significance of clinical factors such as substance misuse and psychopathic personality disorder have been highlighted (Monahan and Appelbaum 2000). However violent risk prediction is an inexact science (Dolan and Doyle 2000) with most studies showing only modest predictive accuracy (Monahan 1994). A number of risk assessment rating scales have been devised in North American settings (see chapter 9) and these need validation elsewhere, including within the UK. It has been suggested that the accuracy of these measures could be enhanced by employing additional physiological measures, assessments of neurocognitive function, and measures of how the individual processes emotional information (Dolan and Doyle 2000).

Predicting treatment response

Other promising developments concern methods for improving prediction of response to treatment. Although there have attempts to systematically investigate the clinical profiles associated with response to biological treatments for disorders such as depression (Stahl 2000), it is fair to say that in practise clinicians rarely if ever employ semi-objective methods such as rating scales to decide what treatment to prescribe. Thus during the 1960s there emerged a broad acceptance that an 'endogenous' pattern of symptoms (guilt, early morning waking, diurnal mood variation diminished libido and weight loss) was a reasonable predictor of good response to tricyclic antidepressants. However this did not prevent this group of drugs being prescribed to depressed subjects without such a profile and indeed 'non endogenous' or 'reactive' depression often responded to tricyclics. The introduction of newer antidepressants such as the serotonin reuptake inhibiters (SSRIs) that have fewer side effects seems actually to have reduced interest in making a global prediction of treatment response. Instead decisions on prescribing are often based on particular symptoms, for example a more sedative drug is prescribed for someone with insomnia or an admixture of depression and anxiety. Also it is not the case that newer drugs have no side effects, just fewer and less harmful side effects, and the discovery of who gets side effects takes place on a trial and error basis. An area of research that has the potential to change all of this is based on the measurement not of symptoms but of genetic polymorphisms.

The basis of current research in *pharmacogenetics* (or *pharmacogenomics*) in psychiatry is that there are broadly two types of genetic variation that can influence response to medication and development of unwanted effects. These are variations in the genes that encode for the target sites at which drugs have their actions, so-called *pharmacodynamic* effects and genetic variations that affect the rate at which drugs are metabolized or broken down and cleared from the body. The latter are called *pharmacokinetic* effects.

Examples of genes likely to be involved in individual differences in pharmacodynamics are those encoding for dopamine D2 type receptors and serotonin receptors of the type known as 5HT2a, since both these receptor types are known to be important in the mode of action of newer 'atypical' antipsychotic drugs such as clozapine. Although still controversial, there is emerging evidence that dopamine and serotonin receptor genotyping can usefully predict response to treatment with clozapine in schizophrenic patients (Arranz *et al.* 2001).

The Cytochrome P450 (CYP) system of liver enzymes governs the rate of metabolism of a large number of drugs and several of the main components are genetically highly polymorphic. Alleleic variation in the genes for different CYPs leads to individual variation in the rates of metabolism of psychotropic drugs, in particular antidepressants. One of the important enzymes in metabolizing most antidepressants is called CYP2 D6. About 10% of white Europeans have a CYP2 D6 genotype that makes for slower breakdown of antidepressants. Individuals who are slow metabolizers are likely to suffer more severe side effects from their medication, and may be less able to tolerate doses that are usually considered necessary to effect clinical improvement. Such individuals may require a much-reduced dose of the drug or alternatively may fare better with a drug that is not metabolized via CYP2 D6. There are also much rarer individuals who are very rapid metabolizers and who may show poor therapeutic response because they do not achieve an adequate blood level on conventional doses.

Therefore, although pharmacogenomics is at present at an early stage, it seems reasonable to envisage a time when treatments are tailored to individuals on the basis of a genetic profile of their likely pharmacokinetic and pharmacodynamic responses. In addition to tailoring of treatments, a major current interest of the pharmaceutical industry is in genomics as a route to new drug discovery. To date most successful treatments for psychopathology have been discovered by chance or by producing chemical variations on the theme of earlier compounds. Using gene mapping methods and positional cloning as mentioned earlier can lead to the discovery of the genes involved, even those involved in complex common disorders. It then becomes feasible to take a *functional genomics* approach that involves studying the variation in the protein structure or levels of expression that is associated with various genetically influenced psychopathologies. This in turn will identify targets at which novel compounds can be directed. Thus it is possible to foresee the development not just of tailored treatments but of specifically targeted treatments.

Conclusions

In some chapters, we have taken a fairly detailed look at the past, in order to demonstrate how the present position has been reached. In this chapter we have tried to look forward and have highlighted some the future directions for research that will require careful attention to the measuring of psychopathology. A recurring theme throughout this book, and one that will not go away, is how to accommodate the dual nature of most forms of psychopathology. Sometimes categories are better descriptors for practical purposes, but nearly always there are dimensional aspects. Doubtless some of the apparent discrepancies between major epidemiological studies in the USA (Regier *et al.* 1998) reflect the problems of selecting cut points on underlying continua.

Although we have emphasized that current classification schemes are provisional and have noted the promise of current highly active areas such as brain imaging and genetics, we do not envisage that either will result in diagnostically useful tests, or that research results will drastically alter the broad shape of current diagnostic groupings. Cognitive psychology, on the other hand, may escape from the laboratory and into the clinic and provide new and useful ways of assessing and treating conditions such as schizophrenia and childhood autism. Arguably this is already happening in the case of depressive and anxiety disorders in that cognitive therapy, embodying a demonstrably successful set of treatment strategies, has a range of theoretical and experimental underpinnings that inform us about why, as well as how it works.

Neuroimaging and genetics are however the joint royal routes to understanding the neurobiological substrata of psychopathology and, as such, offer potential benefits in exploring and developing rational biological treatments. In particular there is a real prospect that pharmacogenomics will have a major impact on drug discovery as well as on providing individually tailored treatment regimes.

Better understanding of causation and improved treatment should result in an improved public image of mental disorder, but there remains considerable public stigma for those who experience mental disorders. Such individuals have been misunderstood, and have often suffered from poor health care in under-resourced services. As we outlined at the beginning of this chapter, there have been improvements in some areas. However, we owe it to those who agree to participate in our research studies, to employ the best methodologies currently available. We hope that we have clearly indicated that one of the key components of best practice must be the inclusion of careful attention to the measurement of psychopathology.

Appendix

Websites for further information

SCID (chapter 5)

http://cpmcnet.columbia.edu/dept/scid
Columbia University website for the Structured Clinical Interview for DSMIV (SCID-I) and related interviews. Site includes details of training, translations, revisions and background reliability and validity studies for SCID-I (see chapter 5), SCID-II (see chapter 9) and KID-SCID (see chapter 8). Order forms for SCID materials can also be downloaded.

ICD10 and SCAN (chapters 3 and 5)

http://www.who.int/msa/scan
World Health Organization website for the *International Classification of Diseases* 10th edition, and the Schedules for Clinical Assessment in Neuropsychiatry (SCAN). The home page includes general information about SCAN, some Powerpoint slides relating to SCAN, a listing of SCAN training centres and a User's Guide. The interview and CATEGO5 scoring program can also be downloaded free, but is password protected. Only those who have completed a training course in the interview are provided with the password.

CIDI and CIDI-auto (chapter 5)

http://www.who.int/msa/cidi/cidisf.htm (CIDI)
http://www.crufad.unsw.edu.au/cidi/cidi.htm (CIDI-auto)
The WHO web sitefor CIDI parallels that for SCAN and provides details of training centres, a literature review and a slide show as well as the instrument itself. A password is required for access.

The Australian site for the CIDI-auto provides a comprehensive account of the computerized version of CIDI. Details for purchasing the program are given.

DIGS, FIGS and SSAGA (chapters 5 and 8)

http://zork.wustl.edu

Website for Washington University St Louis Missouri USA, with links to the National Institute of Mental Health, National Institute of Drug Abuse, National Institute of Addiction and Alcohol Abuse and the Alzheimer's Disease Genetic Consortium web sites. The Diagnostic Interview for Genetic Studies (DIGS), Family Interview for Genetic Studies (FIGS) (see chapter 5) and the Semi-Structured Assessment for Genetics of Alcoholism (SSAGA) (see chapter 8) can be obtained although a password is required before interviews can be downloaded. Hard copies of the interviews can be purchased from the site.

OPCRIT and Hypescheme (Chapter 6)

http://www.iop.kcl.ac.uk/IoP/Departments/SGDPsy/opcrit.stm
http://www.iop.kcl.ac.uk/IoP/Departments/SGDPsy/hypescheme.stm

Website for the Social Genetic and Developmental Psychiatric Research Centre, at the Institute of Psychiatry in London, for further details about the OPCRIT and Hypeschemes packages. Both are available free of charge.

Bibliography

Abou-Saleh, M. T., Ghubash, R., Daradkeh, T. K. (2001) Al Ain Community Psychiatric Survey. I. Prevalence and socio-demographic correlates. *Social Psychiatry and Psychiatric Epidemiology* 36(1): 20–38.

Achenbach, T. M., Edelbrock, C. S. (1978) Classification of child psychopathology: A review and analysis of imperical efforts. *Psychological Bulletin* 85: 1275–1301.

Aertgeerts, B., Buntinx, F., Ansoms, S., Fevery, J. (2001) Screening properties of questionnaires and laboratory tests for the detection of alcohol abuse or dependence in a general practice population. *British Journal of General Practice* 51(464): 172–173.

Albert, M., Cohen, C. (1992) The test for severe impairment: an instrument for the assessment of patients with severe cognitive dysfunction. *Journal of American Geriatrics Society* 40(5): 449–453.

Albrecht, G., Veerman, J. W., Damen, H., Kroes, G. (2001) The child behaviour checklist for group care workers: a study regarding the factor structure. *Journal of Abnormal Child Psychology* 29(1): 83–89.

Alexopoulos, G. S., Abrams, R. C., Young, R. C., Shamoran, C. A. (1988) Cornell Scale for Depression in Dementia. *Biological Psychiatry* 23: 271–284.

Allen, N. H. P., Burns, A. B. (1995) The non-cognitive features of dementia. Review in *Clinical Gerontologist* 5: 57–75.

Allen, N. H., Gordon, S., Hope, T., Burns, A. (1997) Manchester and Oxford University Scale for the psychopathological assessment of dementia. *International Psychogeriatrics* 9 (suppl. 1): 131–136.

Aman, M. G., Tasse, M. J., Rojahn, J., Hammer, D. (1996) The Nisonger CBRF: A for children with developmental disabilities. Research in Developmental Disabilities child behaviour rating form. *Research in Developmental Disabilities* 17: 41–57.

Ambrosini, P. J. (2000) Historical developments and present status of the schedule for affective disorders and schizophrenia for school age children (K-SADS) *Journal of the American Academy of Child and Adolescent Psychiatry* 39(1): 49–58.

American Psychiatric Association (1968) *Diagnostic and Statistical Manual,* 2nd edn. American Psychiatric Association, Washington DC.

American Psychiatric Association (1980) *Diagnostic and Statistical Manual of Mental Disorders*, 3rd edn. American Psychiatric Association, Washington DC.

American Psychiatric Association (1987) *Diagnostic and Statistical Manual of Mental Disorders*, 3rd revised edn. American Psychiatric Association, Washington DC.

American Psychiatric Association (1994) *Diagnostic and Statistical Manual of Mental Disorders*, 4th edn. American Psychiatric Association, Washington DC.

Ancill, R. J., Rogers, D., Carr, A. C. (1985) Comparison of computerised self-rating scales for depression with conventional observer ratings. *Acta Psychiatrica Scandinavica* 71(3): 315–317.

Andreasen, N. C., Flaum, M., Ardut, S. (1987) The Comprehensive Assessment of Symptoms and History (CASH). An instrument for assessing diagnosis and psychopathology. *Archives of General Psychiatry* 49(8): 615–623.

Andreasen, N. C., Olsen, S. (1982) Negative and positive schizophrenia. Definition and validation. *Archives of General Psychiatry* 39(7): 789–794.

Andreasen, N. C, Olsen, S. A., Dennert, J. W., Smith, M. R. (1982) Ventricular enlargement in schizophrenia: relationship to positive and negative symptoms. *American Journal of Psychiatry* 139: 297–302.

Andreasen, N. C., Flaum, M., Swayze, V. W., Tyrrell, G., Arndt, S. (1990) Positive and negative symptoms in schizophrenia. A critical reappraisal. *Archives of General Psychiatry* 47(7): 615–621.

Andrews, G., Slade, T., Peters, L. (1999) Classification in psychiatry. ICD10 versus DSMIV. *British Journal of Psychiatry* 174: 3–5.

Angold, A. (2000) Assessment in child and adolescent psychiatry, in M. G. Gelder, J. J. Lopez-Ibor and N. C. Andreasen (eds) *New Oxford Textbook of Psychiatry*. Oxford University Press, Oxford.

Angold, A., Prendergast, M., Cox, A., Harrington, R., Simonoff, E., Rutter, M. (1995) The child and adolescent psychiatric assessment. *Psychological Medicine* 25(4): 739–753.

Ansseau, M., Doumont, A., Cerfontainne, J. L., Charles, G., Mirel, J. (1982) The necessity for standardised diagnosis in research in biological psychiatry. Attempted integration of research diagnostic criteria into the AMDP system. *Acta Psychiatrica Belgica* 82(4): 422–440.

Araya R., Rojas, G., Fritsch, R., Acuma, J., Lewis, G. (2001) Common mental disorders in Santiago, Chile: Prevalence and socio-demographic correlates. *British Journal of Psychiatry* 178: 228–233.

Armand, W., Loranger, A. W., Sarytorius, N., Andreoli, A., Berger, P., Buchheim, P. et al.. (1994) The World Health Organization, Alcohol, Drug abuse, and Mental health administration International Pilot Study of Personality Disorders. *Archives of General Psychiatry* 51: 215–224.

Armitage, P., Berry, G. (1994) *Statistical Methods in Medical Research*, 3rd edn. Blackwell Science, Oxford.

Arranz, M. J., Munro, J., Osborne, S., Collier, D., Kerwin, R. W. (2001) Applications of pharmacogenetics in psychiatry. *Expert Opinion in Pharmacotherapy* 2(4): 537–542.

Asberg, M., Schalling, D. (1979) Construction of a new psychiatric rating instrument, the Comprehensive Psychopathological Rating Scale (CPRS) *Progress in Neuro-Psychopharmacology* 3(40): 405–12.

Auer, S. R., Scian, S. G., Yassce, R. A., Reisberg, B. (1994) The neglected half of Alzheimer's disease: cognitive and functional concomitance of severe dementia. *Journal of American Geriatrics Society* 42: 1266–1272.

Aylward, E., Burt, D., Thorpe, L., Lia, F., Dalton, A. J. (1997) Diagnosis of dementia with individuals with intellectual disability: Report of the Task-force for development of the criteria for diagnosis of dementia in individuals with mental retardation. *Journal of Intellectual Disability Research* 41: 152–64.

Azevedo, M. H., Soares, M. J., Coelho, I., Dourado, A., Valente, J., Macedo, A. *et al.* (1999) Using consensus OPCRIT diagnoses. An efficient procedure for best estimate life-time diagnoses. *British Journal of Psychiatry* 175: 154–157.

Bauman, L. J. (1994) Mental health of inner city mothers of children with chronic conditions. Presented at the Ambulatory Paediatric Association Annual Meeting, Seattle, Washington.

Baron, M., Asnis, L., Gruen, R. (1981) The Schedule for Schizotyal Personalities (SSP): A diagnostic interview for schizotypal features. *Psychiatry Research* 4: 213–228.

Bech, P. (1984) The instrumental use of rating scales for depression. *Pharmacopsychiatry* 17(1): 22–28.

Bech, P., Coppen, A. (1990) *The Hamilton Scales*. Psychopharmacology Series 9. Springer Verlag, New York.

Beck, A. T., Ward, C. H., Mendelson, M., Mock, J., Erbaugh, J. (1962) Reliability of psychiatric diagnoses: 2. A study of the consistency of clinical judgements and ratings. *American Journal of Psychiatry* 119: 351–357.

Beck, A. T., Ward, C. H., Mendelson, M., Mock, J., Erbaugh, J. (1961) An inventory for measuring depression. *Archives of General Psychiatry* 4: 561–71.

Beck, A. T., Guth, D., Steer, R. A., Ball, R. (1997) Screening for major depression disorders in medical inpatients with the Beck Depression Inventory for Primary Care. *Behaviour Research and Therapy* 35(8): 785–91.

Bentall, R. P., Claridge, G. S., Slade, P. D. (1990) The multi-dimensional nature of schizotypal traits: a factor analytic study with normal subjects. *British Journal of Clinical Psychology* 28(4): 363–367.

Bifulco, A., Bernazzani, O., Moran, P. M., Ball, C. (2000) Lifetime stress/or current depression: preliminary findings of the Adult Life Phase Interview (ALPHI) *Social Psychiatry and Psychiatric Epideminology* 35(6): 264–275.

Black, K., Peters, L., Rui, Q., Milliken, H., Whitehorn, D., Kopala, L. C. (2001) Duration of untreated psychosis predicts treatment outcome in an early psychosis program. *Schizophrenia Research* 47(2–3): 215–222.

Blandford, G. F. (1888) Classification of insanity in R. Quain (ed.) *A Dictionary of Medicine*. Longmans and Co, London.

Blessed, G., Tomlinson, B. E., Roth, M. (1968) The association between quantitative measures of dementia and of senile change in cerebral grey matter of elderly subjects. *British Journal of Psychiatry* 114: 797–811.

Bleuler, E. (1950) Dementia praecox or the group of schizophrenias (1911) trans. S.M Clemens. Yale University Press, New Haven and London.

Bobon, D., Mormont, C., Doumont, A., Mirel, J., Bonhomme, P., Ansseau, M. *et al.* (1982) Factor analysis of the French revision of the AMDP rating scales. *Acta Psychiatrica Belgica* 82(4): 374–389.

Boyle, M. H., Offord, D. R., Racine, Y. A., Fleming, J. E. (1993) Evaluation of the revised Ontario Child Health Study Scales. *Journal of Child Psychology and Psychiatry and Allied Disciplines* 34(2): 189–213.

Boyle, M. H., Offord, D. R., Racine, Y. A., Szatmari, P., Sanford, M., Fleming, J. E. (1996) Interviews versus check lists: adequacy for classifying childhood psychiatric disorder based on adolescent reports. *International Journal of Methods in Psychiatric Research* 6(4): 309–19.

Brebion, G., Gorman, J. M., Malaspina, D., Sharif, Z., Amador, X. (2001) Clinical and cognitive factors associated with verbal memory task performance in patients with schizophrenia. *American Journal of Psychiatry* 158(5): 758–764.

Bridgman, P. W. (1927) *The Logic of Modern Physics*. New York, Macmillan.

Brindle, D. (2000) Taking the lead in *The Guardian Society* 25 October 2000.

Broadhead, W. E., Leon, A. C., Weissman, M. M., Barrett, J. E., Blacklo, R. S., Gilbert, T. T. *et al.* (1995) Development and validation of the SDDS-PC screen for multiple mental disorders in primary care. *Archives of Family Medicine* 4: 211–19.

Brockington, J. F., Kendell, R. E., Leff, J. P. (1978) Definitions of schizophrenia: concordance and prediction of outcome. *Psychological Medicine* 8: 387–98.

Brodman, K., Erdman, A. J., Lorge, I., Wolff, G., Broadbent, T. H. (1949) The Cornell Medical Index: An adjunct to the medical interview. *Journal of the American Medical Association* 140: 530–45.

Brown, G. W., Harris, T. O. (1978) *Social Origins of Depression. A Study of Psychiatric Disorder in Women*, 5th edn. Routledge, London.

Brown, R. L. (1992) Identification and office management of alcohol and drug disorders, in M. F. Fleming and K. L. Barry (eds) *Addictive Disorders*. Mosby Year Book, St Louis.

Brugha, T. S., Bebbington, P. E., Jenkins, R. (1999a) A difference that matters: comparisons of structured and semi-structured psychiatric diagnostic interviews in the general population. *Psychological Medicine* 29(5): 1013–1020.

Brugha, T. S., Bebbington, P. E., Jenkins, R., Meltzer, H., Taub, N. A., Janas, M. *et al.* (1999b) Cross validation of a general population survey diagnostic interview: a comparison of CIS-R with SCAN ICD-10 diagnostic categories. *Psychological Medicine* 29(5): 1029–1042.

Bucks, R. S., Ashworth, D. L., Wilcock, G. K., Seigfried, K. (1996) Assessments of activities of daily living in dementia: development of the Bristol Activities of Daily Living Scale. *Age and Ageing* 25: 113–120.

Burns, A. B., Jacobi, R., Levy, R. (1990) Psychiatric phenomena in Alzheimer's disease: disorders of thought content. *British Journal of Psychiatry* 157: 72–76.

Burton, R. (1652) *Anatomy of Melancholy.*

Butcher, J. N. (1990) *Development and use of the MMPI-2 content scales.* University of Minnesota Press, Minneapolis.

Byrne, L. M., Wilson, P. M. A., Bucks, R. S., Hughes, A. O., Wilcock, G. K. (2000) The sensitivity to change over time of the Bristol Activities of Daily Living Scale in Alzheimer's disease. *International Journal of Geriatric Psychiatry* 15: 656–661.

Cahn, C. H. (1999) DSM classification in H. Freeman (ed.) *A Century of Psychiatry.* Harcourt, London.

Cappeliez, P., Quintal, M., Blouin, M., Gagne, S., Bourgeois, A., Finlay, M. *et al.* (1996) Psychometric properties of the French version of the Modified Mini-Mental State (3MS) in a sample of patients seen in geriatric psychiatry. *Canadian Journal of Psychiatry* 41(2): 114–121.

Cardno, A. G., Jones, L. A., Murphy, K. C., Sanders, R. D., Asherson, P., Owen, M. J. *et al.* (1999) Dimensions of psychosis in affected sibling pairs. *Schizophrenia Bulletin* 25(4): 841–50.

Carney, M. W. P., Roth, M., Garside, R. F. (1965) The diagnosis of depressive syndrome and the prediction of ECT response. *British Journal of Psychiatry* 111: 659–74.

Caron, C., Rutter, M. (1991) Comorbidity in child psychopathology: concepts, issues and research strategies. *Journal of Child Psychology and Psychiatry* 32: 063–1080.

Carpenter, W. T., Strauss, J. S., Bartko, J. J. (1973) Flexible system for the diagnosis of schizophrenia: a report from the WHO pilot study of schizophrenia. *Science* 182: 1275–1278.

Carroll, B. J., Feinberg, M., Smouse, P. E., Rawson, S.G., Greden, J. F. (1981) The Carroll Rating Scale for Depression. Development, reliability and validation. *British Journal of Psychiatry* 138: 194–200.

Cattell, R. B. (1956) Validation and intensification of the sixteen personality factor questionnaire. *Journal of Clinical Psychology* 12: 205–214.

Cattell, R. B. (1973) *Personality and Mood by Questionnaire.* Jossey-Bass, San Francisco.

Cerel, J., Fristad, M. A. (2001) Scaling structured interview data: a comparison of two methods *Journal of the American Academy of Child and Adolescent Psychiatry* 40(3): 341–346.

Chalder, T., Berelowitz, G., Pawlikowska, T., Watts, L., Wessely, S., Wright-Wallace, E. P. (1993) Development of a fatigue scale. *Psychosomatic Research* 37(2): 147–153.

Chambers, W., Puig-Antich, J., Hirsch, M. (1985) The assessment of the affective disorders in children and adolescent by semi-structured interview. Test reliability of the K-SADS-P. *Archives of General Psychiatry* 24: 696–702.

Cicchetti, D. (1984) The emergence of developmental psychopathology. *Child Development* 55: 1–7.

Cicchetti, D., Cohen, D. (eds) (1995) *Developmental Psychopathology.* Wiley, New York.

Cloninger, C. R. (1994) Temperament and personality. *Current Opinions in Neurobiology* 4: 266–273.

Cloninger, C. R. (1987) A systematic method for clinical description and classification of personality variants. *Archives of General Psychiatry* 44: 573–588.

Cloninger, C. R., Svrakic, D. M., Przybeck, T. R. (1993) A psychobiological model of temperament and character. *Archives of General Psychiatry* 50: 975–990.

Cohen, J. A. (1960) A coefficient of agreement for normal scales. *Educational and Psychological Measurements* 20: 37.

Condon, J. T., Corkindale, C. J. (1997) The assessment of depression in the postnatal period: a comparison of four self-report questionnaires. *Australian and New Zealand Journal of Psychiatry* 31(3): 353–359.

Conners, C. K. (1998) Rating scales in attention deficit/hyperactivity disorder: used in assessment and treatment monitoring. *Journal of Clinical Psychiatry* 59: 24–30.

Conners, C. K., Sitarenios, G., Parker, J. D., Epstein, J. N. (1998) The revised Conners' Parent Rating Scale (CPRS-R): factor structure reliability and criterion validity. *Journal of Abnormal Child Psychology* 26(4): 257–68.

Cooper, J. (1999) ICD-10: mental disorders chapter of The International Classification of Diseases, tenth revision, pp. 302–6 in *A Century of Psychiatry* (ed. H. Freeman). London: Mosby-Wolfe.

Copeland, J. R. M., Dowey, M. E., Wood, N., Searle, R., Davidson, I. A., McWilliam, C. (1987) Range of mental illness among the elderly in the community: prevalence in Liverpool using the GMS-AGECAT package. *British Journal of Psychiatry* 150: 815–823.

Costa, P. T., McCrae, R. R. (1992) *Revised NEO Personality Inventory (NEO-PI-R) and NEO Five–Factor Inventory (NEO-FFI): Professional Manual.* Odessa, FL: Psychological Assessment Resources.

Costello, C. G. (1992) Research on symptoms versus research on syndromes. Argument in favour of allocating more time to the study of symptoms. *British Journal of Psychiatry* 160: 304–309.

Costello, E. J., Angold, A. (1985) Scales to assess child and adolescent depression: check-lists, screens, and nets. *Journal of the American Academy of Child and Adolescent Psychiatry* 27(6): 726–737.

Costello, E. J., Edelbrock, C. S., Costello, A. J. (1985) Validity of the NIHM diagnostic interview schedule for children: a comparison between psychiatric and pediatric referrals. *Journal of Abnormal Child Psychology* 13(4): 579–595.

Costello, H., Moss, S., Prosser, H., Hatton, C. (1997) Reliability of the ICD 10 version of the Psychiatric Assessment Schedule for Adults with Developmental Disability (PAS-ADD). *Social Psychiatry, Psychiatric Epidemiology* 32(6): 339–343.

Cottler, L. B., Robins, L. N., Grant, B., Blaine, J., Altamura, A. C., Andrews, G. *et al.* (1991) The CIDI-CORE substance abuse and dependence questions: cross cultural and nosological issues. *British Journal of Psychiatry* 159: 653–659.

Cottler, L. B., Robins, L. N., Helzer, J. E. (1989) The reliability of CIDI-SAM: a comprehensive substance abuse interview. *British Journal of Addiction* 84(7): 801–814.

Cox, J. L., Holden, J. M., Sagovsky, R. (1987) Detection of post natal depression. The development of the 10 item Edinburgh post natal depression scale. *British Journal of Psychiatry* 150: 782–786.

Craddock, N., Asherson, P., Owen, M. J., Williams, J., McGuffin, P., Farmer, A. E. (1996) Concurrent validity of the OPCRIT diagnostic system: comparison of OPCRIT diagnoses with consensus best estimate lifetime diagnoses. *British Journal of Psychiatry* 169: 1–6.

Craig, T. J., Jandorf, L., Rubinstein, J. (1995) Interrater and observer/ self-report correlation of psychopathology in routine clinical practice. *Clinical Psychiatry* 7(1): 25–31.

Crammer, J. L. (1996) Training and education in British psychiatry 1770–1970 in H. Fring and G. E. Berrialls (eds) *150 Years of British Psychiatry,* vol. 2. Athlone, London.

Crow, T. J. (1980) The molecular pathology of schizophrenia: more than one disease process. *British Medical Journal* 280: 66–68.

Cummins, J. L., Megar, M., Gray, K. *et al.* (1994) The neuro psychiatric inventory. *Neurology* 44: 2308–2314.

Cunningham-Owens, D. (1999) Neuroimaging in H. Freeman (ed.) *A Century of Psychiatry,* vol. 2. Harcourt, London.

Curran, S., Newman, S., Taylor, E., Asherson, P. (2000) Hypescheme: an operational criteria checklist and minimum dataset for molecular genetic studies of attention deficit and hyperactivity disorders. *American Journal of Medical Genetics (Neuropsychiatric Genetics)* 96(3): 244–250.

Davidson, R., Bunting, B., Raistrick, D. (1989) The homogeneity of the alcohol dependence syndrome: a factorial analysis of the SADD questionnaire. *British Journal of Addiction* 84: 907–915.

Deary, I. J., Peter, A., Austin, E., Gibson, G. (1998) Personality traits and personality disorders. *British Journal of Psychology* 89(4): 647–661.

Deb, S., Braganza, J. (1999) Comparison of ratings scale for the diagnosis of dementia in adults with Down's syndrome. *Journal of Intellectual Disability Research* 43(5): 400–407.

DeForge, B. R., Sobal, J. (1988) Self report depression scales in the elderly: the relationship between the CES-D and Zung. *International Journal of Psychiatry in Medicine* 18(4): 325–338.

DiLalla, D. L., Gottesman, I. I., Carey, G., Bouchard, T. J. (1996) Heritability of the MMPI personality indicators of psychopathology in twins reared apart. *Journal of Abnormal Psychology* 105(4): 491–499.

Dohrenwend, D. P., Yager, T. S., Egri, G., Mendelson, F. S. (1978) The Psychiatric Status Schedule as a measure of dimensions of psychopathology in general population. *Archives of General Psychiatry* 35: 731–737.

Dolan, M., Cox, D. N., Hare, R. D. (1995) *The Hare Psychopathy Checklist–Revised Screening Version (PCL:SV)*. Toronto, Multi-Health Systems.

Dolam, M., Douglas, K. S., Eaves, D. (1997) Assessing risk of violence to others in C. D. Webster and M. A. Jackson (eds) *Impulsivity: Theory, Assessment and Treatment*. Guilford Press, New York.

Dolan, M., Doyle, M., Quinsey, V. L. (1993) Violent recidivism of mentally disordered offenders: the development of a statistical prediction instrument. *Criminal Justice and Behaviour* 20: 315–335.

Dolan, M., Doyle, M. (2000) Violence risk prediction. Clinical and actuarial measures and the role of the psychopathy checklist. *British Journal of Psychiatry* 177: 303–312.

Doraiswamy, P. M., Kaiser, L. (2000) Variability of the Mini-Mental State examination in dementia. *Neurology* 54(7): 1538–1539.

Doumont, A., Charles, G., Mirel, J., Thiry, D., Ansseau, M. (1982) Comparability between the AMDP scales and the Research Diagnostic Criteria for the diagnosis of endogenous depression. *Acta Psychiatrica Belgica* 82(4): 413–421.

Dowson, J. H. (1992) Assessment of DSM-III-R personality disorders by self-report questionnaire: the role of informants and a screening test for co-morbidity personality disorders (STCPD). *British Journal of Psychiatry* 161: 344–352.

Drummond, D. C. (1990) The relationship between alcohol dependence and alcohol related problems in a clinical population. *British Journal of Addiction* 85: 357–366.

Dunn, G. (1999) *Statistics in Psychiatry*. Arnold, London.

Dyce, J. A. (1997) A big five factors of personality and their relationship to personality disorders. *Journal of Clinical Psychology* 53(6): 587–593.

Dyson, V., Appleby, L., Altman, E., Doot, M., Luchins, D. J., Delehan, M. (1998) Efficiency and validity of commonly used substance abuse screening instruments in public psychiatric patients. *Journal of Addictive Diseases* 17(2): 57–76.

Edwards, B. C., Lambert, M. J., Moran, P. W., McCully, T., Smith, K. C., Ellingson, A. G. (1984) A meta-analytic comparison of the Beck Depression Inventory and the Hamilton Rating Scale for Depression as measures of treatment. *British Journal of Clinical Psychology* 23(2): 93–9.

Einfield, S. I., Tonge, V. J. (1992) *Manual for the Developmental Behavioural Check List*. Monash University Centre for Developmental Psychiatry and School of Psychiatry, University of New South Wales.

Einfeld, S. I., Tonge, V. J. (1996) Population prevalence of psychopathology in children and adolescent with intellectual disability. 2: Epidemiological findings. *Journal of Intellectual Disability Research* 40: 99–109.

Erdman, H. P., Klein, M. H., Griest, J. H., Skare, S. S., Husted, J. J., Helzer, J. E. *et al.* (1992) A comparison of two computer-administered versions of the NIMH Diagnostic Interview Schedule. *Journal of Psychiatric Research* 26(1): 85–95.

Erikson, K. (1964) Notes on the sociology of deviance in H. Becker (ed.) *The Other Side*. The Free Press, New York.

Esquirol, J. E. D. (1833) *Observations of the Allusions of the Insane*. Renshaw and Rush, London.

Evenhuis, H. M. (1992) Evaluation of a screening instrument for dementia in ageing mentally retarded persons. *Journal of Intellect Disability Research* 36(4): 337–347.

Everitt, B. S. (1996) *Making Sense of Statistics in Psychology*. Oxford University Press, Oxford.

Ewing, A. (1984) Detecting alcoholism. The CAGE questionnaire. *Journal of the American Medical Association* 252: 1905–1907.

Eysenck, H. J. (1960) *The Structure of Human Personality*. New York, MacMillan; London, Methuen.

Eysenck, H. J., Eysenck, S. B. (1963) *Eysenck Personality Inventory*. University of London Press, London.

Eysenck, H. J., Eysenck, S. B. (1975) *Manual of the Eysenck Personality Inventory*. Hodder and Stoughton, London.

Fahrer, R., Antonucci, T. C., Gagnon, M. *et al.* (1992) Depressive symptomatology and cognitive functioning: an epidemiological survey in an elderly community sample of France. *Psychological Medicine* 22: 159–172.

Fairburn, C. G., Cooper, Z. (1993) The eating disorder examination in C. G. Fairburn and G. T. Wilson (eds) *Binge Eating: Nature Assessment and Treatment*, 12th edn. Guilford Press, New York.

Farmer, A. E., Chubb, H., Jones, I., Hillier, J., Smith, A., Borysiewicz, B. (1996) Screening for psychiatric morbidity in subjects presenting with chronic fatigue syndrome. *British Journal of Psychiatry* 168: 354–358.

Farmer, A. E., Cosyns, P., Le Eoyer, M., Maier, W., Morse, O., Sargeant, M. *et al.* (1993) A SCAN-SADS comparison study of psychotic subjects and their first degree relatives. *European Archives of Psychiatry and Clinical Neuroscience* 242(6): 352–357.

Farmer, A. E., Harris, T., Redman, K., Sadler, S., Mahmood, A., McGuffin, P. (2000) Cardiff Depression Study. A sib-pair study of life events and familiality in major depression. *British Journal of Psychiatry* 176: 150–155.

Farmer, A. E., Jenkins, P. J., Katz, R., Ryder, L. (1991) A comparison of CATEGO derived ICD VIII and DSM- III classification using the composite international diagnostic interview in severely psychiatrically ill subjects. *British Journal of Psychiatry* 158: 177–183.

Farmer, A. E., Jones, I., Williams, J., McGuffin, P. (1993) Defining schizophrenia: operational criteria. *Journal of Mental Health* 2: 209–222.

Farmer, A. E., Katz, R., McGuffin, P., Bebbington, P. (1987) A comparison of the composite diagnostic interview (CIDI) and the present state examination (PSE) *Archives of General Psychiatry* 44: 1064–1068.

Farmer, A. E., McGuffin, P., Gottesman, I. I. (1985) Searching for the split in schizophrenia: a twin study perspective. *Psychiatry Research* 13: 109–118.

Farmer, A. E., McGuffin, P., Spitznagel, E. L. (1983) Heterogeneity in schizophrenia: a cluster analytic approach. *Psychiatry Research* 8: 1–12.

Farmer, A. E., McGuffin, P., Spitznagel, E. L. (1983) A cluster analytic approach to schizophrenia. *Schizophrenia Research.*

Farmer, A. E., Wessely, S., Castle, D., McGuffin, P. (1992) Methodological issues in using a polydiagnostic approach to define psychotic illness. *British Journal of Psychiatry* 161: 824–830.

Fava, G. A., Kellner, R., Munari, F., Pavan, L. (1982) The Hamilton Depression Rating Scale in normals and depressives. *Acta Psychiatrica Scandinavica* 66(10): 26–32.

Fava, G. A., Kellner, R., Lisansky, J., Park, S., Perini, G. I., Zielezyn, M. (1986) Rating depression in normals and depressives:observer versus self-rating scales. *Journal of Affective Disorders* 11(1): 29–33.

Feighner, J. P., Robins, E., Guze, S. B., Woodruffe, R. A., Winokur, G., Munoz, R. (1972) Diagnostic criteria for use in psychiatric research. *Archives of General Psychiatry* 26: 57–67.

Feinberg, M., Carroll, B. J., Smouse, P. E., Rawson, S. G. (1981) The Carroll rating scale for depression. III. Comparison with other rating scales. *British Journal of Psychiatry* 138: 205–209.

First, M. B., Spitzer, R. L., Gibbon, M., Williams, J. B. W., Benjamin, L. (1994) *Structured Clinical Interview for DSMIV Axis-II Personality Disorders (SCID-II version 2.0)*. Biometrics Research Department, New York Psychiatric Institute, New York.

Fish, F. (1974) Clinical psychopathology. In *Signs and Symptoms in Psychiatry* M. Hamilton (ed.). Wright, Bristol.

Folstein, M. F., Folstein, S. E., McHugh, P. R. (1975) Mini mental state: a practical method for grading the cognitive state of patients for the clinician. *Journal of Psychiatric Research* 2: 189–198.

Frances, A. (1982) Categorical and dimensional systems of personality diagnosis: a comparison. *Comprehensive Psychiatry* 23(6): 516–527.

Fraser, W. (2000) Introduction: an age of enlightenment in M. G. Gelder, J. J. Lopez-Ibor and N. C. Andreasen (eds) *New Oxford Textbook of Psychiatry*. Oxford Univerity Press.

Freeman, B. J., Ritvo, E. R., Yokota, A., Ritvo, A. (1986) A scale for rating symptoms of patients with the syndrome of autism in real life settings. *Journal of American Academic Child Psychiatry* 25(1): 130–136.

Freud, S. (1895) On the grounds for detaching a particular syndrome from neuras-thenia, under the description 'anxiety neurosis' in the standard edition of *The Complete Psychological Works of Sigmund Freud*, vol. 3, J. Strachey (ed.). Hogarth Press, London.

Freud, S. (1904) The psychopathology of every day life in the standard edition of *The Complete Psychological Works of Sigmund Freud*, vol 6, J. Strachey (ed.). Hogarth Press, London.

Fugita, S. S., Crittenden, K. S. (1990) Towards culture and population specific norms for self-reported depressive symptomatology. *International Journal of Social Psychiatry* 36(2): 83–92.

Garner, D. M. (1991) *Eating Disorder Inventory*, vol. 2. Psychological Assessment Resources, Odessa , Florida.

Garner, D. M., Garfinkel, P. E. (1979) The eating attitudes test. An index of the symptoms of anorexia nervosa. *Psychological Medicine* 9: 273–279.

Ghubash, R., Daradkeh, T. K., Al Naseri, K. S., Al Bloushi, N. B., Al Daheri, A. M. (2000) The performance of the Center for Epidemiological Study Depression Scale (CES-D) in an Arab female community. *International Journal of Social Psychiatry* 46(4): 241–249.

Glass, A. U. (1978) Psychiatric screening in a medical clinic. *Archives of General Psychiatry* 35: 1189–1195.

Goldberg, D. P. (1981) Estimating the prevalence of a disorder from the results of a screening test in J. K. Wing., P. Bebbington and L. Robins (eds) *What is a Case?* Grant McIntyre, London.

Goldberg, D. P. (1972) *The Detection of Psychiatric Illness by Questionnaire, Maudsley Monograph no. 21.* Oxford University Press, Oxford.

Goldberg, D. P., Blackwell, B. (1970) Psychiatric illness in general practise. A detailed study using a new method of case identification. *British Medical Journal* 1(707): 439–443.

Goldberg, D. P., Cooper, B., Eastwood, M. R., Kedward, H. B., Shepherd, M. (1970) A standardised psychiatric interview for use in community surveys. *British Journal of Preventative Social Medicine* 24(1): 18–23.

Goldberg, D. P., Huxley, P. (1992) *Common Mental Disorders: a Bio-social Model.* Tavistock/Routledge, London.

Goldberg, D. P., Mann, A., Tylee, A. (2000) Psychiatry in primary care in M. G. Gelder, J. J. Lopez-Ibor and N. C. Andreasen (eds) *New Oxford Textbook of Psychiatry.* Oxford University Press.

Goldberg, D. P., Sharp, D., Nanayakkara, K. (1995) The field trial of the mental disorders section of ICD-10 designed for primary care. *Family Practice* 12: 466–473.

Goldberg, D. P., Williams, P. (1988) *User's Guide to the General Health Questionnaire.* NFER-Nelson, Windsor.

Goldberg, L. R. (1992) The development of markers for the big-five factor structure. *Psychological Assessment* 4: 26–42.

Goodman, R. (1997) The strengths and difficulties questionnaire: a research note. *Journal of Child Psychology and Psychiatry and Allied Disciplines* 38(5): 581–586.

Gottesman, I. I., Shields, J. (1972) *Schizophrenia, a thin study vantage point.* Academic Press, London.

Gottlieb, G. L., Gur, R. E., Gur, R. C. (1988) Reliability of psychiatric scales in patients with dementia of the Alzheimer's type. *American Journal of Psychiatry* 145(7): 857–860.

Griffin, P. T., Kogout, D. (1988) Validity of orally administered Beck and Zung Depression Scales in a state hospital setting. *Journal of Clinical Psychology* 44(5): 756–759.

Guelfi, J. D. (1988) Standardised clinical evaluation of depressive and anxious symptomatology. *Clinical Neuropharmacology* 11(12): S59–68.

Gurin, G., Veroff, J., Feld, S. (1960) *Americans View their Mental Health.* Basic Books, New York.

Hachinski, V. C., Iliff, L. D., Zilka, E., Du Boulay, G. H., McAllister, V. L., Marshall, J. *et al.* (1975) Cerebral blood flow in dementia. *Archives of Neurology* 32: 632–637.

Hamilton, M. (1959) The assessment of anxiety states by rating. *British Journal of Medical Psychology* 32: 50–55.

Hamilton, M. (1960) A rating scale for depression. *Journal of Neurology, Neurosurgery and Psychiatry* 23: 56–62.

Hamilton, M. (1967) The development of a scale for primary depressive illness. *British Journal of Social and Clinical Psychology* 6: 278–296.

Handwerk, M. L., Friman, P. C., Larzelere, R. (2000) Comparing the DISC and youth self-report. *Journal of the American Academy of Child and Adolescent Psychiatry* 39(7): 807–808.

Hanley, J. A., McNeil, B. J. (1983) A method for comparing the areas under receiver operating characteristic curves derived from the same cases. *Radiology* 148: 839–843.

Hare, E. (1990) Old familiar faces: some aspects of the asylum era in Britain in R. M. Murray and T. H. Turner (eds) *Lecturers on the History of Psychiatry: The Squibb Series*. Gaskell, London.

Hare, R. D. (1991) *Manual for the Hare Psychopathy Checklist-Revised*. Toronto, Multi-Health Systems.

Harris, B., Huckle, P., Thomas, R., John, S., Fung, H. (1989) The use of rating scales to identify post-natal depression. *British Journal of Psychiatry* 154: 813–817.

Harris, G. T., Rice, M. E., Quinsey, V. L. (1993) Violent recidivism of mentally disordered offenders: the development of a statistical prediction instrument. *Criminal Justice and Behaviour* 20: 315–335.

Harrison, B., Huckle, P., Thomas, R., Johns, S., Fung, H. (1989) The use of rating scales to identify post natal depression. *British Journal of Psychiatry* 154: 814–817.

Hart, S. D., Cox, D. N., Hare, R. D. (1995) *The Hare Psychopathy Checklist-Revised Screening Version (PCL-SV)*. Multi-Health Systems, Toronto.

Harvey, P. D., Neale, J. M. (1983) The specificity of thought disorder to schizophrenia: research methods in their historical perspective in B. Mahler (ed.) *Progress in Experimental Personality Research*, vol. 12. Academic Press, New York.

Hathaway, S. R., McKinley, J. C. (1967) *The MMPI Manual* (Revised Edition). Psychological Corporation, New York.

Hecker, E. (1871) Die Hebephrenie. *Virchows Archiv fur Pathologische Anatomie* 52: 392–449.

Helmes, E., Reddon, J. R. (1993) A perspective on developments in assessing psychopathology: a critical review of the MMPI and MMPI-2. *Psychological Bulletin* 113(3): 453–471.

Helzer, J. E., Robins, L. N., Kroughan, L. N., Welner, A. (1981) Renard diagnostic interview. Its reliability and procedural validity with physicians and lay interviewers. *Archives of General Psychiatry* 38(4): 393–398.

Hempel, C. G. (1961) Introduction to problems of taxonomy in J. Zubin (ed.) *Field Studies in the Mental Disorders*. Grune and Stratton, New York.

Hill, P. (1997) Child and adolescent psychiatry in R. Murray, P. Hill and P. McGuffin (eds) *The Essentials of Postgraduate Psychiatry*, 3rd edn. Cambridge University Press.

Hills, H. A. (1995) Diagnosing personality disorders: An examination of the MMPI-2 and MCMI-II. *Journal of Personality Assessment* 65(1): 21–34.

Hodges, K. (1993) Structured interviews for assessing children. *Journal of Child Psychological Psychiatry* 34(1): 49–68.

Hodges, K., McKnew, D., Cytryn, L., Stern, L., Kline, J. (1982) The Child Assessment Schedule (CAS) diagnostic interview: a report on reliability and validity. *Journal of American Academic Child Psychology* 21(5): 468–473.

Holland, A. J. (2000) Classification and diagnosis psychiatric assessment and needs assessment in M. G. Gelder, J. J. Lopez-Ibor and N. C. Andreasen (eds) *New Oxford Textbook of Psychiatry*. Oxford University Press, Oxford.

Hope, T., Fairburn, C. G. (1992) The Present Behavioural Examination (PBE): the development of an interview to measure current behavioural abnormalities. *Psychologie Medicale* 22(10): 223–230.

Hopko, D. R., Averill, P. M., Small, D., Greenlee, H., Varner, R. V. (2001) Use of the Brief Psychiatric Rating Scale to facilitate differential diagnosis at acute inpatient admission. *Journal of Clinical Psychiatry* 62(4): 304–312.

Housefield, G. N. (1973) Computerised transverse axial scanning (tomography): Part 1: descriptions of the system. *British Journal of Radiology* 46: 1016–1022.

Hughes, C. W., Rintelmann, J., Emslie, G. J. Lopez, M., MacCabe, N. (2001) A revised version of the BPRS-C for childhood psychiatric disorders. *Journal of Child and Adolescent Psychiatry* 11(1): 77–93.

Huxley, A., Prasher, V. P., Haque, M. S. (2000) The dementia scale for Down's syndrome. *Journal of Intellect Disability Research* 44(6): 697–698.

Hyler, S. E., Skodal, A. E., Oldham, J. M., Kellman, H. D., Doidge, N. (1992) Validity of the Personality Diagnostic Questionnaire – revised: a replication in an outpatient sample. *Comprehensive Psychiatry* 33(2): 73–77.

Ilfeld, F. W. (1976) Further validation of a psychiatric symptom index in a normal population. *Psychological Reports* 39: 1215–1228.

International Human Genome Sequencing Consortium (2001) Initial sequencing and analysis of the human genome. *Nature* 409: 860–921.

Jablensky, A. (1999a) The conflict of the nosologists: views on schizophrenia and manic depressive illness in the early part of the twentieth century. *Schizophrenia Research* 39(2): 95–100.

Jablensky, A. (1999b) The nature of psychiatric classification: issues beyond ICD-10 and DSM-IV. *Australian and New Zealand Journal of Psychiatry* 33(2): 137–144.

Jablensky, A. (1997) The 100-year epidemiology of schizophrenia. *Schizophrenia Research* 28: 111–125.

Jablensky, A., Hugler, H., von Cranach, M., Kalinov, K. (1993) Kraepelin revisited: a reassessment and statistical analysis of dementia praecox and manic depressive insanity in 1908. *Psychological Medicine* 23: 843–858.

Jaspers, K. (1963) *General Psychopathology,* trans. from 7th edn by J. Hoenig and M. W. Hamilton. Manchester University Press, Manchester.

Jenkins, R. (1997) Comprehensive nosology and health. Presentation at the American Psychiatric Association Meeting held in Toronto May 1997. (Abstract no. 32B)

Jenkins, R., Lewis, G., Bebbington, P., Brugha, T., Farrell, M., Gill, B. *et al.* (1997) The National Psychiatric Morbidity survey of Great Britain initial findings from the household survey. *Psychological Medicine* 27(4): 775–789.

John, O. P., Caspi, A., Robbins, R. W., Moffitt, T. E., Stouthaner-Loeber, M. (1994) The Little Five: exploring the normological network of the five-factor model of personality in adolescent boys. *Child Development* 65: 160–178.

John, O. P, Donahue, E. M., Kentle, R. L. (1991) *The Big Five Inventory – Versions 4a and 54* (technical report). Institute of Personality and Social Research, University of California, Berkeley, CA.

John, O. P., Srivastava, S. (1999) The Big Five trait taxonomy: history, measurement and theoretical perspectives in L. A. Pervin and O. P. John (eds) *Handbook of Personality: Theory and Research.* Guilford Press, New York.

Johnson, J., Weissman, W. W., Klerman, G. L. (1992) Service utilisation and social morbidity associated with depressive symptoms in the community. *Journal of the American Medical Association* 267: 1478–1483.

Jones, L. A., Cardno, A. G., Murphy, K. C., Sanders, R. D., Gray, M. Y., McCarthy, G., McGuffin, P., Owen, M. J., Williams, J. (2000) The King schizotypy questionnaire as a quantitative measure of schizophrenia liability. *Schizophrenia Research* 45: 213–221

Jung, C. G. (1923) *Psychological Types* trans. H. G. Baynes. Routledge Kegan Paul, London.

Kahlbaum, K. L. (1874) *Catatonia* (trans.1974) John Hopkins University Press, Baltimore.

Kaufer, D. I., Cummings, J. L., Ketchel, P., Smith, V., Macmillan, A., Shelley, T. *et al.* (2000) Validation of the NPI-Q, a brief clinical form of the neuropsychiatric inventory. *Journal of Neuropsychiatry and Clinical Neurosciences* 12(2): 233–239.

Kaufman, J., Birmaher, B., Brent, D., Rao, U., Flynn, C., Moreci, P. *et al.* (1997) Schedule for Affective Disorders and Schizophrenia for school-age children – Present and Lifetime version (K-SADS-PL): initial reliability and validity data. *Journal of American Academy of Child Adolescent Psychiatry* 36(7): 980–988.

Kay, S. R., Fiszbein, A., Opler, L. A. (1987) The Positive And Negative Syndrome Scale (PANSS) for schizophrenia. *Schizophrenia Bulletin* 12(2): 261–276.

Kay, S. R., Opler, L. A., Spitzer, R. L., Williams, J. B., Fiszbein, A., Gorelick, A. (1991) SCID-PANSS: a two tier diagnostic system for psychotic disorders. *Comprehensive Psychiatry* 32(4): 355–361.

Kay, S. R., Sevy, S. (1990) Pyramidal model of schizophrenia. *Schizophrenia Bulletin* 16: 537–545.

Kendell, R. E. (1982) The choice of diagnostic criteria for biological research. *Archives of General Psychiatry* 39: 1334–1339.

Kendell, R. E. (1975) *The Role of Diagnosis in Psychiatry*. Blackwell Science Publications, Oxford.

Kendler, K. S. (1990) Towards a scientific psychiatric nosology: strengths and limitations. *Archives of General Psychiatry* 47: 969–973.

Kendler, K. S., Lieberman, J. A., Walsh, D. (1989) The Structured Interview for Schizotypy (SIS): s preliminary report. *Schizophrenia Research* 12: 81–88.

Kessler, R. C., McGonagle, K. A., Zhao, S., Nelson, C. B., Hughes, M., Eshleman, S. *et al.* (1994) Lifetime and 12 month prevalence of DSM-IIIR psychiatric disorders in the United States: results from the National Co-morbidity Survey. *Archives General Psychiatry* 51: 8–19.

Knesevich, J. W., Biggs, J. T., Clayton, P. J., Ziegler, V. E. (1977) Validity of the Hamilton Rating Scale for Depression. *British Journal of Psychiatry* 131: 49–52.

Komitz, A. A., Jackson, H. J., Judd, F. K., Cockram, A. M., Kyrios, M., Yeatman, R. *et al.* (2001) A comparison of the Composite International Diagnostic Interview (CIDI-auto) with the clinical assessment in diagnostic mood and anxiety disorders. *Australian and New Zealand Journal of Psychiatry* 35(2): 224–230.

Kovacs, M. (1981) Rating scales to assess depression in school aged children. *Acta Paedopsychiatrica* 46(5–6): 305–315.

Kraepelin, E. (1896) Der psychologische Versuch in der Psychiatrie. *Psycholog Arbeit* 1.

Kraepelin, E. (1913) *Psychiatrie*, vol. 3, part 2, trans. as *Dementia Praecox and paraphenia*. Livingstone, Edinburgh.

Kramer, M. (1961) Some problems for international research suggested by observations as differences in first admission rates to mental hospitals of England and Wales, and of the United States. *Proceedings of the Third World Congress of Psychiatry* 3: 153–160.

Kraupl Taylor, K. F. (1971) A logical analysis of the medico-psychological concept of disease: Part I. *Psychological Medicine* 1: 356–364.

Kretschmer, E. (1936) *Physique and Character*, 2nd edn, trans. W. J. H. Sprott and K. P. Trench. Trubner, New York.

Lamberts, H., Woods, M. (1987) *International Classification of Primary Care.* Oxford, Oxford University Press.

Lamberts, H., Magruder, K., Jathol, B. R. G., Pincus, H., Okkes, I. (1998) The classification of mental disorders in primary care: a guide through a difficult terrain. *International Journal of Psychiatry in Medicine* 28(2): 159–176.

Langfeldt, G. (1939) *The Schizophrenic States.* E. Munksgaard, Copenhagen.

Lasa, L., Ayuso-Mateos, J. L., Vazquez-Barquero, J. L., Diez-Marique, F. J., Dowick, C. F. (2000) The use of the Beck Depression Inventory to screen for depression in the general population: a preliminary analysis. *Journal of Affective Disorders* 57: 261–265.

Lebert, F., Pasquier, F., Souliez, L., Petit, H. (1998) Fronto-temporal Behavioural Scale. *Alzheimer's Disease and Associated Disorders* 12(4): 335–339.

Leckman, J. F., Sholomskas, D., Thompson, W. D., Belanger, A.,Weissman, M. M. (1982) Best estimate of lifetime psychiatric diagnosis: a methodological study. *Archives of General Psychiatry* 39(8): 879–883.

Lee, D. T., Wong, C. K., Ungvari, G. S., Cheung, L. P., Haines, C. J., Chung, T. K. (1997) Screening psychiatric morbidity after miscarriage: application of the 30-item General Health questionnaire and the Edinburgh Postnatal Depression Scale. *Psychosomatic Medicine* 59(2): 207–210.

Lehman, A. F. (1996) Measures of quality amongst persons with severe and persistent mental disorders in G. Thornicroft and M. Tansella (eds) *Mental Health Outcome Measures.* Springer Verlag, Heidelberg.

Leouffre, P. J., Tempier, R., Dongier, M. H. (1990) The diagnosis of alcoholism in family medicine: a pilot study of the correlation of the Michigan Alcoholism Screening Test and the level of serum gamma-glutyltransferase. *Canadian Medical Association Journal* 143(6): 504–506.

Leon, A. C., Olfson, M., Weissman, M. M., Portera, L. (1996) Evaluation of screens for mental disorders in primary care. *Psychopharmacological Bulletin* 32(2): 352–361.

Leopold, N. A., Borson, A. J. (1997) An alphabetical 'WORLD': a new version of an old test. *Neurology* 49(6): 1521–1524.

Lewis, G., Pelosi, A. J., Araya, R., Dunn, G. (1992) Measuring psychiatric disorder in the community: a standardised assessment for use by lay interviewers. *Psychological Medicine* 22(2): 465–486.

Lewis, G., Pelosi, A. J., Glover, E., Wilkinson, G., Stansfeld, S. A., Williams, P., Shepherd, M. (1988) The development of a computerised assessment for minor psychiatric disorders. *Psychological Medicine* 18(3): 737–745.

Liddle, P. F. (1987) The symptoms of chronic schizophrenia: a re-examination of the positive – negative dichotomy. *British Journal of Psychiatry* 151: 145–151.

Lippman, S., Manshadi, M., Christie, S., Gultekin, A. (1987) Depression in alcoholics by the NIMH-Diagnostic Interview Schedule and Zung Self-rating Depression Scale. *International Journal of the Addictions* 22(3): 273–281.

Lorr, M., Klett, C. J., McNair, D. M. (1963) *Syndromes of Psychosis*. Pergamon Press, Oxford.

Loranger, A. W., Sartorius, N., Andreoli, A., Berger, P., Buchheim, P., Channabasavanna, S. M. *et al.* (1994) The World Health Organisation, Alcohol, Drug Abuse and Mental Health Administration, international pilot study of personality disorders. *Archives of General Psychiatry* 51: 215–224.

Luby, J. L., Svrakic, D. M., McCallum, K., Przybeck, T. R., Cloninger, T. R. (1999) The junior Temperament and Character inventory: preliminary validation of a child self-report measure. *Psychology Reports* 84: 1127–1138.

Lykouras, L., Oulis, P., Adrachta, D., Daskalopoulou, E., Kalfakis, N., Triantaphyllou, N. *et al.* (1998) Beck Depression Inventory in the detection of depression among neurological inpatients. *Psychopathology* 31(4): 213–219.

McCrae, R. R., Costa, P. T. (1999) A five factor theory of personality in L. A. Pervin and O. P. John (eds) *Handbook of Personality*, 2nd edn. New York: Guilford Press.

McGuffin, P., Farmer, A. E., Gottesman, I. I. (1987) Is there really a split in schizophrenia? The genetic evidence. *British Journal of Psychiatry* 150: 581–592.

McGuffin, P., Farmer, A. E., Harvey, I. (1991) A polydiagnostic application of operational criteria in studies in psychotic Illness: Development and reliability of OPCRIT system. *Archives of General Psychiatry* 48: 764–770.

McGuffin, P., Martin, N. (1999) Behaviour and genes. *British Journal of Medicine* 319: 37–40.

McGuffin, P., Owen, M. J., Farmer, A. E. (1995) The genetic basis of schizophrenia. *The Lancet* 346: 678–682.

McGuffin, P., Riley, B., Plomin, R. (2001) Genomics and behaviour. Towards behavioural genomics. *Science* 291(5507): 1232–1249.

McLellan, A. T., Luborsky, L., Erdlen, F. R. *et al.* (1980) The Addiction Severity Index: a diagnostic evaluation profile of substance abuse patients in E. Goltheil, A. T. McLellan and K. A. Druley (eds) *Substance Abuse and Psychiatric Illness*. Pergamon Press New York.

McMillan, A. M. (1959) A survey technique for estimating the prevalence of psychoneurotic and related types of disorders in communities in B. Passamanick (ed.) *Epidemiology of Mental Disorders*. New York: American Association for the Advancement of Science, Publication No. 60.

Maher, B. A., Maher, W. B. (1994) Personality and psychopathology: a historical perspective. *Journal of Abnormal Psychology* 103: 72–77.

Maier, W., Heuser, I., Phillip, M., Frommberger, U., Demuth, W. (1988) Improving depression severity assessment II. Content, concurrent and external validity of three observer depression scales. *Journal of Psychiatric Research* 22(1): 13–19.

Maier, W., Minges, J., Lichtermann, D. (1994) Personality variations in healthy relatives of schizophenics. Schizophrenia Research 12: 81–88.

Maier, W., Phillip, M., Heuser, I., Schegal, S., Buller, R., Wetzel, H. (1988) Improving depression severity assessment I. Reliability, internal validity and sensitivity to change of three observer depression scales. *Journal of Psychiatric Research* 22(1): 3–12.

Manchander, R., Hirsch, S. R., Barnes, T. R. E. (1989) A review of rating scales for measuring symptom changes in schizophrenia research in C. Thompson (ed.) *The Instruments of Psychiatric Research*. John Wiley and Sons, Chichester.

Mann, A. H., Raven, P., Pilgrim, J., Khanna, S., Velayudham, A., Suresh, K. P., Channabasavanna, S. M., Janca, A., Sartorius, N. (1999) An assessment of the Standardised Assessment of Personality as a screening instrument for the International Personality Disorder Examination: a comparison of informant and patient assessment for personality disorder. *Psychological Medicine* 29(4): 985–989.

Mannuzza, S., Fyer, A. J., Klein, D. F., Endicott, J. (1986) Schedules for Affective Disorders and Schizophrenia – Lifetime Version modified for the study of anxiety disorders (SADS-LA): rationale and conceptual development. *Journal of Psychiatric Research* 20(4): 317–325.

Matson, J. L., Kazdin, A. E., Senatore, V. (1984) Psychometric properties of the psychopathology instrument for mentally retarded adults. *Applied Research in Mental Retardation* 5(1): 81–89.

Matzner, F. (1997) Preliminary test-retest reliability of the KID-SCID. Scientific Proceedings, American Psychiatric Association Meeting.

Meagher, D., Quinn, J., Murphy, P., Kinsella, A., Mullaney, J., Waddington, J. (2001) Relationship of the factor structure of psychopathology in schizophrenia to the timing of initial intervention with antipsychotics. *Schizophrenia Research* 50(1–2): 95–103.

Meehl, P. E. (1962) Schizotaxia, schizotypy, schizophrenia. *American Psychologist* 17: 827–838.

Menzies, R. J., Webster, C. D., Sepejak, D. S. (1985) The dimensions of dangerousness: Evaluating the accuracy of psychometric predictions of violence among forensic patients. *Law and Human Behaviour* 9: 35–56.

Meyer, A. (1957) Psychobiology (Salman Lectures given in 1932) Charles C Thomas, Springfield, Illinois.

Miller, E. (1996) Twentieth century British clinical psychology and psychiatry: their historical relationship. *Twentieth Century British Clinical Psychology and Psychiatry* 56–170.

Miller, H. C. (1961) Accident neurosis. *British Medical Journal* I: 919–925.

Mojtabai, R., Rieder, R. O. (1998) Limitations to the symptom-orientated approach to psychiatric research. *British Journal of Psychiatry* 173: 198–202.

Monahan, J. (1994) The prediction of violent behaviour towards a second generation of theory and policy. *American Journal of Psychiatry* 141: 10–15.

Monahan, J., Appelbaum, P. S. (2000) Developing a clinical useful actuarial tool for assessing violence risk. *British Journal of Psychiatry* 176: 312–320.

Montgomery, S., Asberg, M. (1979) A new depression scale designed to be sensitive to change. *British Journal of Psychiatry* 134: 382–389.

Monterio, I. M., Boksay, I., Auer, S. R., Torossian, C., Sinaiko, E., Reisburg, B. (1998) Reliability of routine clinical instruments for the assessment of Alzheimer's disease administered by telephone. *Journal of Geriatric Psychiatry and Neurology* 11(1): 18–24.

Moore, J., Farmer, A. E. (2002) Personality and illness in M. Rutter and E. Taylor (eds) *Child and Adolescent Psychiatry*, 3rd edn. Cambridge University Press.

Morey, L. C., Gunderson, J., Quigley, B. D., Lyons, M. (2000) Dimensions and categories: the 'Big Five' factors and the DS personality disorders. *Assessment* 7(3): 203–216.

Moroney, J. T., Bagiella, E., Desmond, D. W., Hachinski, V. C., Moelsae, P. K., Gustafson, L. *et al.* (1997) Meta-analysis of the Hachinski Ischemic Score in pathologically verified dementias. *Neurology* 49(4): 1096–1105.

Morris, J. C. (1993) The Clinical Dementia Rating (CDR): current version and scoring rules. *Neurology* 43: 2412–2414.

Moss, S. C. (1993) Psychiatric morbidity in older people with moderate and severe learning disability (mental retardation) Part I: Development and reliability of the patient interview (the PAS–ADD). *British Journal of Psychiatry* 163: 471–480.

Mullen, P. E. (1997) The mental states of mind in R. Murray, P. Hill and P. McGuffin (eds) *The Essentials of Postgraduate Psychiatry*, 3rd edn. Cambridge University Press, Cambridge.

Munoz, R. F., McQuaid, J. R., Gonzalez, G. M., Dimas, J., Rosales, V. A. (1999) Depression screening in a women's clinic: using automated Spanish- and English-language voice recognition. *Journal of Consulting Clinical Psychology* 67(4): 502–510.

Murden, R. A., Galbraith, J. (1997) A modified Mini-Mental State Exam for use in the poorly educated. *Clinical Gerontologist* 17(4): 23–33.

Murray, H. A. (1943) *Thematic Apperception Test Manual.* Harvard University Press. Cambridge, Mass.

Nakaya, M., Suwa, H., Ohmori, K. (1999) Latent structures underlying schizophrenic symptoms: a five-dimensional model. *Schizophrenia Research* 39: 39–50.

Nasr, S. J., Altman, E.G., Rodin, M. B., Jobe, T. H., Burg, B. (1984) Correlations of the Hamilton and Carroll Depression Rating Scales: A replication study among psychiatric outpatients. *Journal of Clinical Psychiatry* 45(4): 67–168.

Nihara, K., Leland, H., Lambert, N. (1993) *Adaptive Behaviour Scales – Residential and Community*, 2nd edn. Pro-Ed, Austin, Texas.

Noordsy, D. L., O'Keefe, C., Mueser, K. T., Xie, H. (2001) Six month outcomes for patients who switch to olanzepine treatment. *Psychiatric Service* 52(4): 501–507.

Nordin, V., Gillberg, C. (1996) Autism spectrum disorders in children with physical or mental disability or both II. Screening aspects. *Developing Medicine in Child Neurology* 38(4): 314–324.

Nurnberger, J., Blehar, M. C., Kaufmann, C. A., York-Cooler, C., Simpson, S.G., Harkavy-Friedman *et al.* Collaborators from the NIMH Genetic Initiative (1994) Diagnosis Interview for Genetic Studies: rationale, unique features and training. *Archives of General Psychiatry* 51: 849–859.

Nutt, D. J., Law, F. D. (2000) Pharmacological and psychological aspects of drugs of abuse in M. G. Gelder, J. J. Lopez-Ibor and N. C. Adreasen (eds) *New Oxford Textbook of Psychiatry*. Oxford University Press, Oxford.

Oberholzer, E. (1924) Tha application of the interpretation of form to psychoanalysis. *Journal of Nervous and Mental Disease* 60: 225–248.

Okun, A., Stein, R. E. K., Bauman, L. J., Silver, E. J. (1996) Content validity of the Psychiatric Symptom Index, CES-Depression Scale and the State-trait Anxiety Inventory from the perspective of DSM-IV. *Psychological Reports* 79: 1059–1069.

Olwens, D. (1993) Bullying at school: Basic facts and effects of a school based intervention programme. *Journal of Child Psychology and Psychiatry* 35: 1171–1190.

Overall, J. E., Gorham, D. R. (1962) The Brief Psychiatric Rating Scale (BPRS). *Psychological Reports* 10: 799–812.

Panisset, M., Roudier, M., Saxton, J., Boller, S. (1994) Severe Impairment Battery: a neuropsychological test for severely demented patients. *Archives of Neurology* 51(1): 41–45.

Parloff, M. B., Kelman, H. C., Frank, J. D. (1954) Comfort, effectiveness and self-awareness as criteria for improvement in psychotherapy. *American Journal of Psychiatry* 111: 343–351.

Patterson, M. B., Mack, J. L., Neundorfer, M. M., Martin, R. J., Smythe, K. A., Whitehouse, P. J. (1992) Assessment of functional ability in Alzheimer's disease: a review and preliminary report on the Cleveland Scale for activities of daily living. *Alzheimer's Disorder and Associated Disorders* 6: 145–163.

Peirson, A. R., Heuchert, J. W., Thomalia, L., Berk, M., Plein, H., Cloninger, C. R. (1999) Relationship between serotonin and the temperament and character inventory. *Psychiatry Research* 13: 237–265.

Perris, C., Eisemann, M., Von Knorring, L., Perris, H. (1984) Presentation of a sub-scale for the rating of depression and some additional items to the comprehensive psychopathological rating scale. *Acta Psychaitrica Scandinavica* 70(3): 261–274.

Perris, C. (1979) Reliability and validity studies of the Comprehensive Psychopatho-logical Rating Scale (CPRS). *Progress in Neuro-Psychopharmacology* 3(4): 13–21.

Perris, C., Ericsson, U., Jacobsson, L., Lindstrom, H., Perris, H. (1979) Interprofes-sional communicability and reliability of the Comprehensive Psychopathologi-cal Rating Scale (CPRS) as assessed by video-taped interviews. *Acta Psychiatrica Scandinavica* 60(2): 144–148.

Persons, J. B. (1986) The advantages of studying psychological phenomena rather than psychiatric diagnoses. *American Psychologist* 41: 1252–1260.

Peters L., Andrews, G. (1995) The procedural validity of the computerised version of the Composite International Diagnostic Interview (CIDI-auto) in anxiety disorders. *Psychological Medicine* 25(6): 1269–1280.

Pietzcker, A., Gebhardt, R. (1983) Depressive syndromes and scales in the AMDP system. *Acta Psychiatrica Scandinavica supplimentum* 310: 65–84.

Pilgrim J., Mann, A. (1990) Use of the ICD10 version of the Standardised Assessment of Personality to determine the prevalence of personality disorder in psychiatric in-patients. *Psychological Medicine* 20(4): 985–992.

Pilkonis, P. A., Heape, C. L., Proietti, J. M., McDavid, J. D., Pitts, T. E. (1995) The reliability and validity of two structured diagnostic interviews for personality disorders. *Archives of General Psychiatry* 52(12): 1025–1033.

Pincus, H. A., Vettorello, N. E., McQueen, L. E., First, M., Wise, T. N., Zarin, D. *et al.* (1995) Bridging the gap between psychiatry and primary care. The DSM-IV-PC. *Psychosomatics* 36(4): 328–335.

Plomin, R., Caspi, A. (1995) Behavioural genetics and personality in L. A. Pervin and O. P. John (eds) *Handbook of Personality: Theory and Research.* Guilford Press, New York.

Plomin, R., DeFries, J. C., McClearn, G. E., Rutter, M. (1997) *Behavioural Genetics,* 3rd edn. W. H. Freeman and Company, New York.

Plomin, R., Rende, R., Rutter, M. (1991) Quantitative genetics and developmental psychopathology in D. Cicchetti., S.L. Toth and L. Erlbaum (eds) *Internalising and Externalising Expressions of Dysfunction: Rochester Symposium on Developmental Psychopathology,* vol. 2. Hillside, New Jersey.

Porter, R. (1997) *The Greatest Benefit to Mankind.* HarperCollins, London.

Powell, B. J., Penick, E. C., Othmer, E. (1985) The discriminant validity of the psychiatric diagnostic interview. *Journal of Clinical Psychiatry* 46(8): 320–322.

Powers, J. S., Spickard, A. (1984) Michigan Alcoholism Screening Test to diagnose early alcoholism in a general practice. *South Medical Journal* 77(7): 852–856.

Prince, M. (1998) Measurement in psychiatry. *International Review of Psychiatry* 10(4): 264–271.

Pristach, C. A., Smith, C. M., Perkins, C. (1993) Reliability of the Self-administered Alcoholism Screening Test (SAAST) in psychiatric inpatients. *Journal of Addiction Diseases* 12(4): 77–88.

Radloff, L. S. (1977) The CES-D scale: a self-report depression scale for research in general populations. *Applied Psychological Measurement* 1: 385.

Rait, G., Burns, A., Baldwin, R., Morley, M., Chew-Graham, C., St Leger, A. S. (2000) Validating screening instruments for cognitive impairment in older South Asians in the United Kingdom. *International Journal of Geriatric Psychiatry* 15(1): 54–62.

Ramsey, M., Winget, C., Higginson, I. (1995) Review: Measures to determine the outcome of community services for people with dementia. *Age and Ageing* 24: 73–83.

Regier, D. A., Myers, J. K., Krammer, M., Robins, L. N., Blazer, D. G., Hough, R. L. *et al.* (1984) The NIMH epidemiological catchment area of program. Hisotrical context major objectives and study population and charcteristics. *Archives of General Psychiatry* 41(10): 934–941.

Regier, D. A., Narrow, W. E., Rae, D. S., Manderscheid, R. W., Locke, D. Z., Goodwin, F. K. (1993) The de facto US mental and addictive service system: epidemiological catchment area, prospective 1-year prevalence rates of disorders and services. *Archives of General Psychiatry* 50: 85–94.

Regier, D. A., Kaelber, C. T., Rae, D. S., Farmer M., Knauper, B., Kessler, R. C. *et al.* (1998) Instruments for mental disorders. Implications for research and policy. *Archives of General Psychiatry* 55: 109–115.

Reich, W. (2000) Diagnostic interview for children and adolescents (DICA) *Journal of American Academic Child and Adolescent Psychiatry* 39(1): 59–66.

Reich, W., Herjanic, B., Welner, Z., Gandhy, P. R. (1982) Development of a structured psychiatric interview for children: agreement on diagnosis comparing child and parent interviews. *Journal of Abnormal Child Psychology* 10: 325–336.

Reich, W., Cottler, L., McCallum, K., Corwin, D., VanEerdewegh, M. (1995) Computerized interviews as a method of assessing psychopathology in children. *Comprehensive Psychiatry* 36(1): 40–45.

Reisburg, B., Ferris, S. H., DeLeon, M. J. *et al.* (1982) The Global Deterioration Scale for assessment of primary degenerative dementia. *American Journal of Psychiatry* 139: 1136–1139.

Reisburg, B., Borenstein, J., Salob, S. P., Ferris, S. H., Franssen, E., Georgotas, A. (1987) Behavioural symptoms in Alzheimer's disease: phenomenology and treatment. *Journal of Clinical Psychiatry* 48(5): 9–15.

Remmington, M., Tyrer, P. J., Newson-Smith, J., Cicchetti, D. V. (1979) Comparative reliability of categorical and analogue rating scales in the assessment of psychiatric symptomatology. *Psychological Medicine* 9(4): 765–770.

Reynolds, C. R., Richmond, B. O. (1997) What I think and feel: a revised measure of children's manifest anxiety. *Journal of Abnormal Child Psychology* 25(1): 15–20.

Richter, P., Werner, J., Heerlein, A., Kraus, A., Saur, H. (1998) On the validity of the Beck Depression Inventory. A review. *Psychopathology* 31(3): 160–168.

Ritchie, C. W., Hayes, D., Ames, D. J. (2000) Patient or client? The opinions of people attending a psychiatric clinic. *Psychiatric Bulletin* 24(12): 447–450.

Roberts, R. E., Solovitz, B. L., Chen, Y. W., Casat, C. (1996) Retest stability of DSM-III-R diagnoses among adolescents using the diagnostic interview schedule for children (DISC-2.1C). *Journal of Abnormal Child Psychology* 24(3): 349–362.

Robins, L. N., Helzer, J. (1986) Diagnostic and clinical assessment: the current state of psychiatric diagnosis. *Annual Review of Psychology* 132: 1187–1192.

Robins, L. N., Helzer, J. E., Croughan, J., Ratcliffe, K. S. (1981) National Institute of Mental Health, Diagnostic Interview Schedule: its history, characteristics and validity. *Archives of General Psychiatry* 38: 381–389.

Robins, L. N., Wing, J., Wittchen, H. U., Helzer, J. E., Babor, T. F., Burke, J. *et al.* (1988) The composite international diagnostic interview: an epidemiological instrument suitable for use in conjunction with different diagnostic systems and in different cultures. *Archives of General Psychiatry* 45: 1069–1077.

Romanoski, A. J., Nestadt, G., Chahal, R., Merchant, A., Folstein, M. F., Gruenberg, E.M. *et al.* (1988) Interobserver reliability of a 'standardised psychiatric examination' for case ascertainment (DSMIII). *Journal of Nervous and Mental Diseases* 176(2): 63–71.

Rosenman, S. J., Korten, A. E., Levings, C. Y. (1997) Computerised diagnosis in acute psychiatry: validity of CIDI-auto against routine clinical diagnosis. *Journal of Psychiatric Research* 35(5): 581–592.

Roth, M., Tym, E., Mountjoy, C. Q., Huppert, F. A., Hendrie, H., Verma, S. *et al.* (1986) CAMDEX. A Standardised Instrument for the Diagnosis of Mental Disorder in the Elderly. *British Journal of Psychiatry* 149: 698–709.

Royal College of Psychiatrists (2001) Diagnostic criteria for psychiatric disorders for use with adults with learning disabilities/mental retardation (DC-LD). Occasional Paper OP48. Gaskell, London.

Russell, G. (2000) Disorders of eating in M. G. Gelder, J. J. Lopez-Ibor and N. C. Andreasen (eds) *The New Oxford Textbook of Psychiatry*. Oxford University Press, Oxford.

Rutter, M., Cox, A., Tupling, C., Berger, M., Yule, W. (1975) Attainment and adjustment into two geographical areas: 1. Prevalence of psychiatric disorder. *British Journal of Psychiatry* 126: 493–509.

Rutter, M. (1988) Epidemiological approaches to developmental psychopathology. *Archives of General Psychiatry* 45: 486–495.

Sandanger, I., Nygard, J. F., Ingebrigtsen, G. (1999) Prevalence, incidence and age of onset of psychiatric disorders in Norway. *Social Psychiatry and Psychiatric Epidemiology* 34(11): 570–579.

Saunders, J. B., Aasland, O. G., Babor, T. F., De la Fuente, J. R., Grant, M. (1993) Development of the Alcohol Use Detection Identification Test (AUDIT) WHO collaborative project on early detection of persons with harmful alcohol consumption. *Addition II* 88: 617–629.

Saxton, J., McGonigle, G., Gibson, K., Swihart, A., Miller, M., Boller, S. (1990) Assessment of the severely impaired patient: description and validation of a neuropsychological test battery. *Psychol Assess* 2: 298–303.

Scadding, J. G. (1967) Diagnosis the clinician and the computer. *Lancet* I: 877–882.

Scheff, T. (1966) *Being Mentally Ill.* Aldine, Chicago.

Schneekloth, T. D., Morse, R.M., Herrick, L. M., Suman, V. J., Offord, K. P., Davis, L. J. (2001) Point prevalence of alcoholism in hospitalised patients: continuing challenges of detection, assessment and diagnosis. *Mayo Clinic Proceedings* 76(5): 457–458.

Schneider, K. (1959) Clinical psychopathology (trans. M. Hamilton) Grune and Stratton. New York.

Schofield, W. (1966) In sickness and in health. *Community Mental Health Journal* 2(3): 244–251.

Schopler, E., Reichler, R. J., DeVillis, R. F., Daly, K. (1980) Toward objective classification of childhood autism: childhood Autism rating scale (CARS) *Journal of Autism Disorder* 10(1): 91–103.

Schriger, D. L., Gibbons, P. S., Langone, C. A., Lee, S., Altshuler, L. L. (2001) Enabling the diagnosis of occult psychiatric illness in the emergency department: a randomized, controlled trial of the computerized, self-administered PRIME-MD diagnostic system. *Annual Emergency Medicine* 37(2): 132–140.

Scian, S. G., Reisburg, B. (1992) Functional Assessment Staging Test (FAST) in Alzheimer's disease: reliability, validity and utility. *Psychogeriatrics* 55: 55–69.

Scott, S. (2000) Developmental psychopathology and classification in childhood and adolescence in M. G. Gelder, J. J. Lopez-Ibor and N. Andreasen (eds) *New Oxford Textbook of Psychiatry.* Oxford University Press.

Seppa, K., Lepisto, J., Sillanaukee, P. (1998) Five shot questionnaire on heavy drinking. *Alcohol Clinical Experience and Research* 22(8): 1788–1791.

Sevin, J., Matson, J. L., Coe, D. A., Fee, V. E., Sevin, B. M. (1991) A comparison and evaluation of three commonly used Autism scales. *Journal of Autistic Developmental Disorders* 21(4): 417–432.

Shaffer, D., Schwab-Stone, M., Fisher, P., Cohen, P., Piacentini, J., Davies, M. *et al.* (1993) The diagnostic interview schedule for children – revised version (DISC-R): I. Preparation, field testing, interrater reliability, and acceptability. *Journal of American Academy Child Adolescent Psychiatry* 32(3): 643–650.

Shaffer, D., Fisher, D., Dulcan, M. K. (1996) The NIMH Diagnostic Schedule for Children version 2.3 (DISC-2.3): Description, acceptability, prevalence rates and performance in the MECA study. *Journal of the American Academy of Child and Adolescent Psychiatry* 35: 865–877.

Shaffer, D., Lucas, C., Richters, J. (1999) *Assessment in Child and Adolescent Psychopathology.* Guilford Press, New York.

Shapiro, M. B., Post, F. (1974) Comparison of self rating of psychiatric patients with ratings made by a psychiatrist. *British Journal of Psychiatry* 125: 36–41.

Shay, K. A., Duke, L. W., Conboy, T., Harrell, L. E., Callaway, R., Folks, D. G. (1991) The clinical validity of the MATTIS Dementia Rating Scale in staging Alzheimer's dementia. *Journal of Geriatric Psychiatry and Neurology* 4(1): 18–25.

Sheldon, W. H., Stevens, S. S., Tucker, W. B. (1942) *The Varieties of Temperament.* Harper, London.

Sims, A. (1988) *Symptoms in the Mind.* Bailliere Tindall, London.

Slezer, M. L., Vinokour, A., van Roojen, L. (1975) A self-administered Short Michigan Alcohol Screening Test (SMAST) *Journal Studies of Alcoholism.* 9: 27–38.

Small, G. W. (1985) Revised Ischemic Score for diagnosing multi-infarct dementia. *Journal of Clinical Psychiatry* 46(12): 514–517.

Snaith, R. P., Constantopoulos, A. A., Jardine, M. Y., McGuffin, P. (1978) A clinical scale for the self-assessment of irritability. *British Journal of Psychiatry* 132: 164–171.

Snaith, R. P. (1996) Present use of the Hamilton Depression Rating Scale: observations on method of assessment in research of depressive disorders. *British Journal of Psychiatry* 168: 594–597.

Sparrow, S., Balla, D., Cicchetti, D. (1984) *Vineland Adaptive Behaviour Scale.* (Interview edition – survey version) American Guidance Association, Circle Pines MN.

Speilberger, C. D. (1983) *State-trait Anxiety Inventory: a Comprehensive Bibliography.* Consulting Psychologists Press, Palo Alto, CA.

Spijker, J., Bijl, R. V., de Graaf, R., Noel, W. A. (2001) Determinants of poor 1 year outcome of DSMIIIR major depression in the general population: results of the Netherlands Mental Health Survey and Incidence Study (NEMESIS). *Acta Psychiatrica Scandinavica* 103(2): 122–130.

Spitzer, R. L. (1966) Mental Status Schedule; potential use as a criterion measure of change in psychotherapy research. *American Journal of Psychiatry* 20(1): 156–167.

Spitzer, R. L., Endicott, J. (1968) DIAGNO: A computer program for psychiatric diagnoses utilising the differential diagnostic procedure. *Archives of General Psychiatry* 18(6): 746–756.

Spitzer, R. L., Endicott, J. R., Robins, E. (1975a) Clinical criteria for psychiatric diagnosis and DSM-III. *American Journal of Psychiatry* 132: 1187–1192.

Spitzer, R. L., Endicott, J. R., Robins, E. (1975b) *Research Diagnostic Criteria: Instrument No.58.* New York State Psychiatric Institute, New York.

Spitzer, R. L., Endicott, J. R., Robins, E. (1978) Research diagnostic criteria: rationale and reliability. *Archives of General Psychiatry* 35: 773–782.

Spitzer, R. L., Endicott, J. R. (1978) *Schedule of Affective Disorders and Schizophrenia*, 3rd edn. Biometrics Research, New York.

Spitzer, R. L., Endicott, J., Cohen, J., Nee, J. (1980) The Psychiatric Status Schedule for epidemiological research. Methodological considerations. *Archives of General Psychiatry* 37(10): 1193–1197.

Spitzer, R. L., Endicott, J., Fleiss, J. L., Cohen, J. (1970) The Psychiatric Status Schedule. *Archive of General Psychiatry* 23(1): 41–55.

Spitzer, R. L., Gilford, L. M. (1968) UPDATE: A computer program for converting diagnoses to the new nomenclature of the American Psychiatric Association. *American Journal of Psychiatry* 125(3): 51–152

Spitzer, R. L., Kronenke, K., Williams, J. B. (1999) Validation and utility of a self report version of PRIME-MD: the PHQ primary care study. Primary care evaluation of mental disorders. Patient health questionnaire. *Journal of the American Medical Association* 282(18): 1733–1744.

Spitzer, R. L., Williams, J. B. W., Gibbon, M., First, M. B. (1992) The Structured Clinical Interview for DSM III R (SCID): history, rationale and description. *Archive General Psychiatry* 49: 624–629.

Spitzer, R. L., Williams, J. B. W., Kroenke, K., Linzer, M., deGruy, F. V., Brody, D. *et al.* (1994) Utility of a new procedure for diagnosting mental disorder in primary care. The PRIME-MD 1000 study. *Journal of the American Medical Association* 272(2): 1749–1756.

Spitznagel, E. L., Helzer, J. E. (1985) A proposed solution to the base rate problem in the caper statistic. *Archives of General Psychiatry* 42(7): 725–728.

Stahl, S. M. (2000) *Essential Psychopharmacology of Depression and Bipolar Disorders.* Cambridge University Press, New York.

Stanger, C., Lewis, M. (1993) Agreement among parents, teachers and children on internalising and externalising behavioural problems. *Journal of Clinical Child Psychology* 22: 107–115.

Stangl, D., Pfohl, B., Zimmerman, M., Bowers, W., Corenthal, C. (1985) A structured interview for the DSMIII personality disorders. A preliminary report. *Archives of General Psychiatry* 42(6): 591–596.

Stein, R. E. K., Jessop, D. J. (1989) Measuring health variables among Hispanic and non-Hispanic children. *Public Health Reports* 104: 377–384.

Stockwell, T., Hodgson, R., Edwards, G. *et al.* (1979) the development of a questionnaire to measure the severity of alcohol dependence. *British Journal of Addiction* 74: 79–87.

Stuart, G. W., Pantelis, C., Klimidis, S., Minas, I. H. (1999) The three syndrome model of schizophrenia: Meta-analysis of an artefact. *Schizophrenia Research* 39: 233–242.

Swets, J. A., Pickett, R.M. (1982) *Evaluation of Diagnostic Systems: Methods for Signal Detection Theory.* Academic Press, New York.

Szasz, T. (1962) *The Myth of Mental Illness*. Secker and Warburg, London.

Taylor, M. A., Abrams, R. (1978) The prevalence of schizophrenia: a reassessment using modern diagnostic criteria. *American Journal of Psychiatry* 135: 945–948.

Taylor, E., Schachar, R., Thorley, G., Wieselberg, M. (1986) Conduct disorder and hyperactivity: I. Separation of hyperactivity and antisocial conduct in British child psychiatric patients. *British Journal of Psychiatry* 149: 760–767.

Tiffany, S. T., Singleton, E., Haertzen, C. A., Henningfield, J. E. (1993) The development of a cocaine craving questionnaire. *Drug and Alcohol Dependence* 34: 19–28.

Tomov, T. (1999) Political abuse of psychiatry in the former Soviet Union in H. Freeman (ed.) *A Century of Psychiatry*. Harcourt, London.

Tonge, B. J., Einfeld, S. I., Krupinski, J. (1996) The use of factor analysis for ascertaining patterns of psychopathology in children with intellectual disability. *Journal of Intellectual Disability Research* 40: 198–207.

Tosnerova, T., Bahbouh, R. (1998) Mini-Mental State Examination: a quick cognitive state test. *Ceskosovenska Psychologie* 42(4): 328–333.

Tsuang, M. T., Winokur, G. (1974) Criteria for subtyping schizophrenia. *Archives of General Psychiatry* 31: 43–47.

Tucker, M. A., Ogle, S. J., Davison, J. G., Eilenberg, M. D. (1987) Validation of a brief screening test for depression in the elderly. *Age and Ageing* 16(3): 139–144.

Tyrer, P. (1990) Diagnosis in personality disorders. *Current Opinion in Psychiatry* 3: 82–187.

Tyrer, P., Cicchetti, D. V., Casey, P. R., Fitzpatrick, K., Oliver, R., Balter, A. *et al.* (1984) Cross-national reliability of a schedule for assessing personality disorder. *Journal of Nervous and Mental Disease* 172(12): 718–721.

Tyrer, P., Owen, R. T., Cicchetti, D. V. (1984) The brief scale for anxiety: a subdivision of the comprehensive psychopathological rating scale. *Journal of Neurology, Neurosurgery and Psychiatry* 47(9): 970–975.

Ustun, T. B., Goldberg, D. P., Cooper, J., Simon, G., Sartorius, N. (1995) A new classification of mental disorders based upon management for use in primary care. *British Journal of General Practice* 45: 211–215.

Ustun, T. B. (1997) Assessment of functioning and the International Classification of Impairment, disabilities and handicaps framework. Abstract (32D) for the American Psychiatric Association Meeting in Toronto.

Venter, J. C., Adams, M. D., Myers, E. W., Li, P. W., Mural, R. J., Sutton, G. G. *et al.* (2001) The sequence of the human genome. *Science* 291: 1304–1351.

Verhulst, F. C., Althaus, M., Berden, G. F. (1987) The child assessment schedule: parent-child agreement and validity measures. *Journal of Child Psychology and Psychiatry* 28(3): 455–466.

Webster, C. D., Douglas, K. S. (1997) Assessing risk and violence to others. In: *Impulsivity: theory, assessment and treatment* (eds. C. D. Webster and M. A. Jackson). Guilford Press, New York.

Wechsler, D. (1992) *Weschsler Intelligence Scale for Children*, 3rd edn. Psychological Corporation, London.

Wechsler, D. (1997) *Weschsler Adult Intelligence Scale*, 3rd edn. Psychological Corporation, Cleveland, Ohio.

Weiner, D. V. (1994) Le geste de pernel: the history of a psychiatric myth in M. S. Micale and R. Porter (eds) *Discovering the History of Psychiatry*. Oxford, Oxford University Press.

Weissman, M. M., Sholomskas, D., Pottenger, M., Prusoff, B. A., Locke, B. Z. (1977) Assessing depressive symptoms in five psychiatric populations: a validation study. *American Journal of Epidemiology* 106(3): 203–214.

Welner, Z., Reich, W., Herjanic, B., Jung, K. G., Amado, H. (1987) Reliability, validity, and parent-child agreement studies of the Diagnostic Interview for Children and Adolescents (DICA). *Journal of American Academic Child and Adolescent Psychiatry* 26(5): 649–653.

Widiger, T. A. (1992) Categorical versus dimensional classification: implications from and for research. *Journal of Personality Disorders* 6(4): 287–300.

Widiger, T. A. (1993) The DSMIIIR categorical personality disorders: a critique and an alternative. *Psychological Inquiry* 4: 75–90.

Widiger, T. A., Frances, A., Spitzer, R. L. (1988). The DSM-III-R personality disorders: an overview. *American Journal of Psychiatry* 145 : 786–795.

Widiger, T. A., Sanderson, C. J. (1995) Towards a dimensional model of personality disorders in DSM-IV and DSM-V in W. J. Livesley (ed.) *The DSM-IV Personality Disorders*. Guilford, New York.

Widiger, T. A., Trull, T. S., Clarkin, J. F., Sanderson, C., Costa, P. T. (1994) A description of the DSM-IIIR and DSM-IV personality disorders with the five-factor model of personality in P. T. Costa and T. A Widigier (eds) *Personality Disorders and the Five-factor Model of Personality*. American Psychiatric Association, Washington DC.

Widiger, T. A., Lynam, D. R. (1998) Psychopathy from the perspective of the five-factor model of personality in T. Million, E. Simonsen, M. Birket-Smith and R. D. Davis (eds) *Psychopathy: Antisocial, Criminal and Violent Behaviour*. Guilford, New York.

Wiersma, D. (1996) Measuring social disabilities in mental health in G. Thornicroft and M. Tansella (eds) *Mental Health Outcome Measures*. Springer Verlag, Herdleberg.

Williams, J., Spurlock, G., McGuffin, P., Mallet, J., Nothen, M. M., Gill, M. *et al.* (1996) Association between schizophrenia and the T 102C polymorphism of the 5-hydroxytryptamine type 2a receptor gene. *The Lancet* 347: 1294–1296.

Williams, J., Farmer, A. E., Ackenheil, M., Kaufmann, C. A., McGuffin, P. (1996b) A multicentre inter-rater reliability study using the OPCRIT computerized diagnostic system. *Psychological Medicine* 26(4): 775–783.

Williams, M. B. (1993) The psychometric properties of schizotypal personality. Unpublished PhD thesis. Institute of Psychiatry, University of London.

Wing, J. K, Babor, T., Brugha, T., Cooper, J., Geil, R., Jablensky, A. *et al.* (1990) SCAN: schedules for the clinical assessment in neuropsychiatry. *Archives of General Psychiatry* 47: 589–593.

Wing, J. K., Bebbington, P., Robins, L. N. (eds) (1981) *What is a Case?* Grant, MacIntyre, London.

Wing, J. K., Cooper, J. E., Sartorius, N. (1974) *The Measurement and Classification of Psychiatric Symptoms.* Cambridge University Press, Cambridge.

Winston, M., Smith, J. (2000) A trans-cultural comparison of four psychiatric case-finding instruments in a Welsh community. *Social Psychiatry, Psychiatric Epidemiology* 35(12): 569–575.

Winter, D. G., Barenbaum, N. B. (1999) History of modern personality theory and research in L. A. Pervin and O. P. John (eds) *Handbook of Personality: Theory and Research.* Guilford Press, New York.

Winter, L. B., Steer, R. A., Jones-Hicks, L., Beck, A. T. (1999) Screening for major depression disorders in adolescent medical outpatients with the Beck Depression Inventory for Primary Care. *Journal of Adolescent Health* 24(6): 389–394.

Wittchen, H.-U., Ustun, T. B., Kessler, R. C. (1999) Diagnosing mental disorders in the community. A difference that matters? *Psychological Medicine* 29(5): 1021–1027

Wittenborn, J. R. (1972) Reliability, validity and objectivity of symptom rating scales. *Journal of Nervous and Mental Diseases* 154(2): 79–86.

Woggon, B. (1979) Comparison between Comprehensive Psychological Rating Scale (CPRS) and the Association for Methodology and Documentation in Psychiatry (AMP) system. *Progress in Neuro-psychopharmacology* 3(4): 423–427.

Woodworth, R. S. (1919) Examination of emotional fitness for warfare. *Psychological Bulletin* 15: 59–60.

World Health Organisation (1973) *Report on International Pilot Study of Schizophrenia,* vol. 1. Geneva, World Health Organisation.

World Health Organisation (1980) *International Classification of Impairments, Disabilities and Handicaps,* 10th revision. Geneva, World Health Organisation.

World Health Organisation (1992) *The ICD-10 Classification of Mental and Behavioural Disorders. Clinical Descriptions and Diagnostic Guidelines.* Geneva, World Health Organisation.

World Health Organisation (1993) *Diagnostic Criteria for Research – Geneva. International Classification of Diseases,* 10th edn. Geneva, World Health Organisation.

World Health Organisation (1996) *Diagnostic and Management Guidelines for Mental Health Disorders in Primary Care ICD-10.* Chapter V, Primary care version. Hogrefe and Huber, Bern.

World Health Organisation International Consortium in Psychiatric Epidemiology (2000) Cross-national comparisons of the prevalences and correlates of mental disorders. *Bulletin of the World Health Organisation* 78(4): 413–426.

Wundt, W. (1903) *Grundzuge der Physiologischen Psychologie,* 5th edn. Leipzig, W. Engelmann.

Young, A. S., Lyons, M. J., Waternaux, C. M., Faraone, S. V., Tsuang, M. T. (1993) The relationship between DSM-III personality disorders and five factor model of personality. *Comprehension of Psychiatry* 34(4): 227–234.

Yule, W. (2000) Developmental psychology through infancy, childhood and adolescence in M. G. Gelder, J. J. Lopez-Ibor and N. C. Andreasen (eds) *New Oxford Textbook of Psychiatry.* Oxford University Press, Oxford.

Yuspeh, R. L., Vanderploeg, R. D., Kershaw, D. A. J. (1998) Validity of a semantically queued recall procedure for the Mini-Mental State examination. *Neuropsychiatry, Neuropsychology and Behavioural Neurology* 11(4): 207–211.

Zigmond, A. S., Snaith, R. P. (1983) The hospital anxiety and depression scale. *Acta Psychiatrica Scandinavica* 67(6): 361–370.

Zimmerman, M. (1994) Diagnosing personality disorders. A review of issues and research methods. *Archives of General Psychiatry* 51(3): 225–245.

Zimmerman, M., Pfohl, B., Stangl, D., Corenthal, C. (1986) Assessment of DSMIII personality disorders: the importance of interviewing an informant. *Journal of Clinical Psychiatry* 47: 261–263.

Zung, W. W. (1990) The role of rating scales in the identification and management of the depressed patient in the primary care setting. *Journal of Clinical Psychiatry* 51: 72–76.

Index

Page numbers in **bold** indicate main discussion.